OVER THE INFLUENCE

Over the Influence

The Harm Reduction Guide to Controlling Your Drug and Alcohol Use

SECOND EDITION

Patt Denning
Jeannie Little

THE GUILFORD PRESS
New York   London

Copyright © 2017 The Guilford Press
A Division of Guilford Publications, Inc.
370 Seventh Avenue, Suite 1200, New York, NY 10001
www.guilford.com

The information in this volume is not intended as a substitute for consultation with healthcare professionals. Each individual's health concerns should be evaluated by a qualified professional.

Printed in the United States of America

This book is printed on acid-free paper.

Last digit is print number: 9   8   7   6   5   4   3   2   1

Library of Congress Cataloging-in-Publication Data is available from the publisher.

ISBN 978-1-4625-2679-6 (paper) — ISBN 978-1-4625-3034-2 (hard)

Artwork by Mariana Spada at Tectonica.

As ever, to our muse, Edith Springer, who led
the first wave of harm reduction in the United States
and never stopped being on fire

To our mentors, Paul Geltner, Alan Marlatt,
and Bob Unger, whose skilled guidance
has kept us attuned to the needs of people
who drink and use drugs

And to our parents, Eileen and Frank
and Jean and Bill, who believed their daughters
could do anything at times and in places where girls
were not supposed to be groundbreakers and leaders

Contents

Purchasers of this book can download and print
enlarged versions of the worksheets at
www.guilford.com/denning2-forms for personal use
or use with clients (see copyright page for details).

Acknowledgments

We were fortunate to work with the same team at The Guilford Press that helped us produce the first edition of *Over the Influence*. Executive editor Kitty Moore is a mover and shaker who, knowing the importance of harm reduction to the American public, spurred us on with her confidence and positive feedback when we just wanted to *do* the work, not spend a year of nights and weekends *writing* about it. Christine Benton is an amazing developmental editor. She provided nonjudgmental critiques and suggestions, sometimes demonstrating that she knows more about our topic than we do! It was her idea to add all of the features that make this edition more usable by people who want to apply harm reduction to their own lives. Rosalie Wieder, our copyeditor, came in at the end and, in microscopic detail, cleaned up inconsistencies and corrected inaccuracies. She even brought back important sentences from the first edition that we had long ago left behind.

Several other people helped us along the way. Center for Harm Reduction Therapy (CHRT) board member Rebecca Pfeiffer-Rosenblum did early data gathering on current drug-use patterns, trauma, substance use, and other important information about why people use drugs. Board member and friend James Pollet, master strategist that he is, reviewed the entire book and helped us rethink and reorder it more coherently. Steve Robitaille, copy writer and friend, helped us find the right words to define harm reduction therapy, guided us to the "bird's-eye" view, and removed unnecessary detail from the Introduction. Our dear friend and colleague Dan Bigg, of the Chicago Recovery Alliance, a founding leader of the harm reduction movement in the United States, reviewed the substance use management chapter and the drug section and supplied essential updates and current perspectives. Finally, our friends Ned Howey and Mariana Spada of Tectonica, the web design company that produces all of our designs, created the awesome graphics throughout the book.

As for the people who keep us going:

Drug users and frontline harm reduction workers tirelessly spread clean needles rather than disease, show love to other drug users by preventing overdose, and always shout out the message that drug users' lives matter. Representing drug users and workers alike, the Harm Reduction Coalition brings the tribe together to exchange ideas, research, and support at blockbuster conferences. They continue to steer a moral course for all of us in the harm reduction movement. The Drug Policy Alliance leads the charge around the world to end the hateful and wasteful War on Drugs, at the same time giving legal counsel to individuals who are caught up in its net.

Increasing numbers of harm reduction psychotherapists and harm reduction–oriented programs offer science-based, compassionate, and pragmatic treatment to active substance users without asking that people change before even beginning treatment. First among them, Andrew Tatarsky of the Center for Optimal Living is our co-leader in developing harm reduction psychotherapy and our leader in promoting it around the world.

Most important, the staff at the CHRT always stay radically client centered, weathering the ups and downs of drinking and drug-using lives, focusing on the good that our clients do, and never rejecting anyone, however risky their substance use. They help us stay true to our belief that *everyone* has the right to self-determination, no matter how much trouble they find themselves in.

Preface

How Did We Get Here?

In 1994, I (Jeannie) was sitting in my first harm reduction group, a group for veterans with posttraumatic stress and other serious emotional problems who also used drugs. This was at a time when people who needed both mental health and drug treatment could find almost no one who would offer both. And no one would offer anything, period, to people who could not or would not quit using drugs, or at least commit to doing so. Outraged, I said, "I'm going to damn well do it myself!" It was the second session of this new group, and a man pushing a shopping cart came in. He was a longtime heroin user who typically spent his days sleeping in waiting rooms and his nights roaming the streets, too afraid to lie down and sleep outside. After settling into a chair, he promptly fell asleep with his head leaning at an awkward angle. At the time this was a no-no (it still is in most places). Sleeping through a group broke all the rules and conventions of group therapy, and the typical response was to ask a person to wake up and participate actively or leave.

Given that I was trying to create something completely different from the usual and customary treatment practices, I decided to focus only on *his* experience, not on anyone else's ideas of right and wrong conduct. He was tired, perhaps nodding out after his morning shot, and he was going to wake up with a crick in his neck. I took my jacket, borrowed a few others, made a pillow, and rested his head on it. The rest of the group was stunned. When they asked why, I answered simply, "Because he is going to wake up with a crick in his neck." The members of this group, which is now more than 20 years old, talked about this episode for a long time. They came to understand that "there but for the grace of God go I. He is better off here than out there somewhere." He was safe, and that made us feel better. They began to create the language of harm reduction: "We are accepted for who we are; we can come as we are; we can say whatever is on our minds; and we understand ourselves better because we have so much freedom here." As one member said, "I only learn what I think when I hear myself talk in this group." The group embraced and fiercely defended the values of kindness, generosity of spirit, acceptance, and trust—trust that people are doing their best, trust that they are making the decisions they need to make in any given moment, and trust that, if they don't show up, it's because they need something else more than they need us today.

Thus began the culture of harm reduction groups, a culture that lives on today in that group and in the dozens, perhaps hundreds, of others that have sprung up in its wake.

★ ★ ★

More than a decade earlier, one day in early 1983, a man walked into the clinic where I (Patt) was working. He was a big guy—or at least it was clear that he *used to be* big. On this day he had some trouble walking down the hall, pausing to catch his breath, and it looked as if his skin was just hanging off him. Steve was only 31, but something was really wrong. What was wrong was that he had AIDS, although neither he, nor his doctors, nor I knew much about it at the time. All we knew was that our patients in the primary care clinic and the attached mental health clinic were dying, quickly and horribly, from mysterious causes. We didn't know what caused AIDS or how it was transmitted. And we certainly didn't have any treatments, let alone a cure. We didn't know if we could catch it from having contact with our patients. Steve was one of 400 patients in our clinic who would eventually die from this disease. But in the meantime, he needed our help.

To cover his fear, Steve did his best to tell jokes and stories about his wild life. He did indeed lead a wild life, not unlike many other gay men at the time. Parties and sex with multiple partners, alcohol and drugs—all part of celebrating gay liberation. But Steve's drugs of choice included far more than most men I worked with: poppers, cocaine, alcohol, marijuana, and "whatever pills someone gives me." Steve brought other issues that complicated his life, drove his substance use, and would challenge my training in how to work with people with mental health and substance use issues.

As I had been taught, I referred Steve to a drug treatment program. A few weeks later he returned to see me. He said that he was "kicked out for being a merry queen," meaning that he didn't quit using drugs and failed every drug test. He talked about feeling humiliated at being told he was an addict, that he couldn't be trusted, and that he had nothing to contribute to his treatment—they knew best, and he could either get with the program or leave.

Alarmed, upset, and angry, I decided to work with Steve myself. For the next 2 years he taught me about himself. He taught me that drug use is often an adaptive response to the powerful force that is grief. He taught me that it is important to ask *why,* to understand people's underlying motivations for using, the benefits that they get, and why they persist despite negative consequences. Steve changed my life. And my work with him during the 3 years before he died began my journey toward harm reduction.

★   ★   ★

Since these moments in our careers, each of us has developed a harm reduction therapy practice. In 2000, we started the Center for Harm Reduction Therapy, where we work with substance users from all walks of life— from successful professionals and entrepreneurs whose drug use is starting to erode their quality of life and relationships to people like Steve and the veteran in Jeannie's group (who later went to rehab, quit using heroin, found a place to live, and started working again for the first time in many years).

Our practice meets drug users where they are, helps them discover *their* desire to change, supports them in many other ways if they choose to change nothing, and *always* moves at their pace. We respect each individual's right, power, and strength to determine the changes he or she wants to make. We and our team of therapists are dedicated to pursuing a deep understanding of our clients so that we can help them create positive outcomes for themselves. We are passionate, flexible, and eternally optimistic.

Over the years, we have worked with thousands of drinkers and drug users in the Bay Area of California, and we have trained thousands of therapists and counselors around the country and in other parts of the world who work with thousands more drug users. But there are millions of drug users in this country, and more than 20 million who *mis*use substances. This book is the best way we know to reach all of you.

Introduction

Why Harm Reduction?

Rebecca walked in and said, "I finally realized why I keep failing out of rehab—I don't want to quit!"

After that announcement and a few jokes, she said she really did want help with her drinking and pot smoking, which was "way too heavy to be good for me." She had already been through three rehabs. Every time, she began smoking and drinking as soon as she got out.

Rebecca had been smoking pot since she was 14 and drinking heavily since her late teens. When we met her, she was smoking every day and bingeing on alcohol every weekend. Well into her 30s, she had picked up a pill habit. She was drinking and driving, had a DUI, and had fallen several times. Her husband and friends were heavy drinkers too, but she "won the prize."

Would it have been tempting to push another rehab? Sure. Was it likely to succeed? Probably not. What Rebecca needed was time and a conducive environment in which to think about her drinking and pot use. She had been putting so much mental and emotional energy into resisting judges', colleagues', and program demands for abstinence, and she was so afraid of a life without intoxication, that she had little room to think dispassionately about herself and her relationship with drugs.

Rebecca needed permission and guidance to explore what it was about her past, her marriage, her job, and her social circle that fueled such excessive drinking. What was her reliance on pot about? And why had she added pills to the mix? She needed encouragement to figure out what she *did* want to do. And, after almost 30 years of heavy substance use, she was going to need practical strategies and skills to put her plan into action. In the meantime, she needed to stay alive and to stop endangering those around her.

Rebecca needed what all people who get into trouble with alcohol and drugs need—understanding, compassion, unbiased information, and options. In our current "Just Say No" culture, and the treatment programs that follow from it, the assumption is that there is only one way, and the only thing we need to understand is that addiction is a disease and all addicts must quit, now and forever, the use of all psychoactive substances. Simple. One size fits all.

Unfortunately, only between 5 and 20% of the 20 or so million people who misuse alcohol and other drugs solve their problems that way. For a myriad of reasons, including that they are not ready or willing to quit, the other 80 to 95% are left, like Rebecca, isolated, alienated, and in danger of incurring or causing serious harm.

Zero tolerance for substance use has not worked, and the jury is *in*. It is no longer considered ethical to deny people access to unbiased information about drugs and to safer drug-using methods. It is no longer considered ethical to segregate drug users from mainstream health care. It is no longer considered ethical to punish drug users for what is a health, not a moral, problem. It is no longer considered ethical to stigmatize drug use. By bringing drug use out into the open, by understanding and not judging, by teaching safety, and by offering options for change that do not box people into corners, harm reduction addresses *all* of the harms that can occur in a drug-using life, regardless of whether a person's use rises to the level of "addiction."

Harm reduction is based on evidence from many sources—academic research into the causes of substance misuse and the mechanisms of change, large surveys of drug use and health, and in-the-field research by hundreds of public health workers. But so-called scientific research is not the only source of evidence. Another important source of information about what works comes from what is called "practice as evidence"—from the observation of the therapists, counselors, case managers, outreach workers, doctors, and nurses who have dedicated their careers to helping people who use drugs. But the *most* important source of evidence for harm reduction comes from the incredible amount of knowledge that drug users have—about drugs and how they work, about how to use them safely, and about what it takes to change a drug-using life.

Whether you realize it or not, *you* have a lot of practice-based evidence. After all, you are the one living with alcohol and other drugs. Harm reduction wants to hear *your* evidence, your lived experience. That way we can put together all of our wisdom to help you deal with the issues that are getting in the way of your living your life the way you want to.

★   ★   ★

This book takes our professional treatment model and translates it for everyday use by anyone who is interested in an alternative approach to substance use and misuse. We reframe old concepts—from *addiction* to a *relationship with drugs,* and from *recovery* to *change.* We aim to help you understand your relationship with alcohol and other drugs so that you can make informed choices that reduce harm in your life and in the lives of those you care about. We invite you to start right where you are, to take your time, and to choose options that will work for *you.*

This is the second edition of this book. Since the first edition in 2004, the United States has reached a tipping point in its relationship with drugs, and people are looking for alternatives to the dominant ideology of abstinence and 12-step "recovery" as the only solutions to their problems with drugs. Harm reduction is seeping into public awareness. Sadly, much of this is the result of the dramatic increase in opioid overdoses, which has sped up access to the life-saving drug naloxone and spurred the passage of "Good Samaritan" laws that protect drug users from arrest if they call 911 when someone overdoses.

In 2004, we did not imagine that drug policy reform would have progressed so far. Needle exchange was illegal under federal law. As was medical marijuana. The federal government just lifted the ban on needle exchange in 2015. Five states and the District of Columbia have legalized marijuana and more are on track to do so. We suspect that, if you are reading this book in 2027, marijuana will be legal all over the country. It will be a legitimate medicine and a legitimate source of recreational intoxication, right alongside alcohol.

There has been an explosion of interest in moderation approaches for alcohol problems, with several well-established programs available in person or online. Even the National Institute of Alcoholism and Alcohol Abuse published a pamphlet, called "Rethinking Drinking," which offers guidelines for moderate drinking. Increasingly, people who use drugs other than alcohol use these programs to moderate their drug use. In harm reduction parlance, they are practicing substance use management.

There has been a resurgence of attention paid to research from the 1960s, '70s, and '80s, research that studied humans' relationship with drugs; research that revealed that most people use drugs in a controlled manner; research that proved that addiction is not just about addictive drugs or diseased people. It is also, some believe, mostly about the circumstances in which we live. A slew of popular new books since 2013 has cast serious doubt on the validity of the disease model of addiction and the neuroscience that claims addiction as a brain disease.

The War on Drugs, which has never succeeded at reducing our use of drugs, is faltering. After 30 years of mass incarceration, devastation in Mexico and Central and South America, and billions of dollars wasted trying to eradicate drugs from the earth, there is no controversy about the fact that the drug war has failed. We are attempting to end mandatory minimum sentencing for drug offenses, equalize sentencing between crack and powder cocaine, and release people from prison for the "crime" of possessing, using, and selling drugs. And federal appeals courts have determined that mandating attendance at AA violates the constitutional separation of church and state.

Portugal has provided us with compelling evidence that ending prohibition makes things far better. In 2001, Portugal, which had the worst heroin problem in Europe, decriminalized the use of all drugs. Far from a mad rush to the nearest heroin dealer, there has been a very small increase in the number of drug *users* and a 50% decrease in opioid *addiction*. In a similar attempt to end the ravages of the illegal drug trade and the endless cycle of imprisonment of its citizens, Uruguay has legalized marijuana.

We have an opportunity to make similar changes in our drug treatment systems. There has already been some change. An increasing number of programs have moved toward a more realistic approach grounded in harm reduction. Harm reduction therapy, the most accessible treatment to date, is poised to be the umbrella for all treatment of substance use and co-occurring disorders in the 21st century. Like our treatment, this book will help you to:

- Understand what drives your use
- Separate the benefits of your drugs from the harms
- Prioritize the issues facing you
- Develop motivation for change
- Implement gradual, realistic steps to achieve your goals
- Take care of yourself while you use
- Applaud your progress

It will also help you explain harm reduction to others and find the right help if you need it.

If you have read *Over the Influence* before, you will find this edition substantially different, not in its attitude and approach but in its presentation. Its focus is less on explaining harm reduction as a new theory and approach and more on the information and techniques you need to apply it to your own life. It offers more self-assessment tools and practical suggestions and is organized so that you can work your way from understanding your drug use to making decisions about how to reduce harm, to putting those changes into effect and evaluating how you're doing. It contains significantly more data. And, in recognition of the fact that we all learn in different ways, it has fewer words and more graphics. You can use this book as a self-help program based on harm reduction therapy or as a source of information and support as you decide on the course of action that's right for you. In this edition we present a lot of material in boxes so that you can read them as desired, using these icons to represent the nature of the content:

 Did You Know . . . ?

 Remember . . .

 More Information

 Self-Reflection

 What the Science Says

Each of you will have preferences for how you like to receive information. As in harm reduction practice, this book gives you options.

★   ★   ★

We have a passion for empowerment and justice and an appreciation for the complexity of each individual's relationship with drugs. This is what drives us.

We believe that people have the right to self-determination.

We believe that drug use is a normal part of human experience.

We believe that people have the right to cope in the best way they can and that it is inhumane to ask someone to give up his or her coping mechanism without offering something to replace it.

We believe that when people have real and unbiased information about drugs, they can and will make informed decisions.

We believe that when people have access to real options for change that are based on evidence, pragmatism, and compassion, they will change more often and more easily.

Finally, we want people to be free—free of punitive sanctions for what they choose to put in their bodies; free of society-induced and program-induced shame and guilt for how they cope; free to study and define their own problems; and free to find solutions that work for them.

We hope that this book will assist you to take control, make decisions, and find your own way. We hope you find that you no longer have to be "under the influence" of drugs *or* "Just Say No" ideology. Rather you can be "over the influence"—a person with the power to learn, to choose, and to change.

1 Welcome to Harm Reduction

Harm reduction is a compassionate and pragmatic approach to helping people resolve their problems with drugs.
—G. Alan Marlatt, eminent researcher in harm reduction, relapse prevention, and mindfulness

Come as you are. These are the first words we say to people who come to us. In other words, you don't have to change a thing. You don't have to promise anything. You don't have to know what you want. You just know you are worried about your drinking or drug use. Or someone else in your life is.

What if people are saying you have to quit? At times that will happen. *You* might be one of the people telling yourself you have to quit! Maybe it's even true. But saying "You have to quit" is akin to saying "Just say no!" Saying it doesn't make it true, and it certainly doesn't make it happen. Hearing "You have to quit" is really just a signal that it's time to start thinking. Research on change tells us that people think and worry before, sometimes *long* before, they act.

In harm reduction, you can be curious, you can be reluctant, you can be confused, you can be mad, or you can be determined. Harm reduction offers a way forward for everyone who wants to understand or do something about his or her drug use. Harm reduction offers . . .

A Different Way of Thinking

Do you know of any doctor who would refuse insulin to a patient with diabetes because he won't stop eating ice cream?

How many heart patients are denied bypass surgery because they still haven't gotten off the couch except to let the dog out, despite their doctor's instructions to get 30 minutes of aerobic exercise a day?

Would a doctor refuse to prescribe oxygen for a patient with emphysema who still smokes?

> Problems with alcohol and drugs are not diseases, crimes, or sins. They are *health issues.*

Doctors who made these unlikely decisions would probably face charges of medical malpractice. Why, then, are people who use or misuse alcohol and other drugs treated differently? People who drink too much or use recreational drugs usually hear "I can't help you until you stop drinking/quit using." That injunction is based on the myth that people cannot solve other problems, including and especially their problems with substances, until they have quit. This makes substance misuse the only "disorder" in the American Psychiatric Association's *Diagnostic and Statistical Manual of Mental Disorders* that requires the sufferer to get rid of his or her symptoms before receiving treatment for the problem!

Until now, both the moral model (manifested in the War on Drugs) and the disease model of addiction have been based on prohibition. They have taken an all-or-

> Harm reduction is realistic and compassionate.

nothing stance toward substance use. Characterized by terms such as "clean" and "dirty" and "in the program" or "out there," one is either an "addict/ alcoholic" who will face "jails, institutions, or death" if he or she keeps using or a "normie" (someone who uses normally, without problems). These terms trap the substance user in a binary identity dilemma and a dichotomous choice to be either an "addict" or "clean and sober."

We disagree with this approach, and that is why we offer you this book.

Harm reduction offers a completely different way of thinking about substance use and misuse. In harm reduction you don't have to choose— harm reduction is a both/and approach to managing drug use and misuse. You can be a daily pot smoker *and* a good parent; a weekend partier *and* a great teacher, lawyer, plumber, or gardener; dependent on heroin *and* a loving partner. You can also have a problem with alcohol and be an occasional cocaine user or heavy meth user and a light pot smoker.

> Harm reduction is a *both/and* instead of an *either/or* philosophy and practice.

Harm reduction takes a health rather than a disease perspective, a compassionate and humane rather than a moralistic and punitive perspective, on why people use drugs and how they get into trouble. It brings substance misuse into the realm of mainstream health care and releases it from the clutches of the criminal justice system and from programs that preach zero tolerance for substance use. Harm reduction is realistic about the fact that, after 45 years and hundreds of billions of dollars, we have made hardly a dent in reducing the use of drugs. In harm reduction practice, drug use and drug problems are understood in the context of each person's overall physical, mental, and emotional health and well-being, not as moral failures, signs of a weak character, a brain disease, or, worst of all, criminal behavior.

From our perspective, you don't have a disease and you certainly are not immoral or weak! Even if you have done bad things while under the influence. Rather, you have a *relationship with drugs*. When we talk about "a relationship with drugs," we mean that *people use drugs for reasons*. Drugs work amazingly well to enhance pleasure, medicate pain, and alter perception. The speed you use does, in fact, get you through the day; alcohol helps you *enjoy* your wife's office holiday party; pot makes conversations more interesting (not to mention its many medical benefits); cocaine was around before Viagra; and heroin takes away *all* the pain. Drugs work; otherwise you wouldn't be using them. Or they did at one time, even if they are now part of a bad habit with which you are stuck. Either way, they are, or have been, a meaningful part of your life. Harm reduction takes that seriously and is *interested* in learning about your relationship with drugs.

Like all relationships, your relationship with drugs is probably complicated—sometimes healthy, sometimes not, sometimes harmless, sometimes disastrous. Like all relationships, it changes over its lifespan. And like all relationships, it takes time and trial and error to change. Harm reduction understands *how* people end up in relationships with drugs, and it recognizes the uniqueness of each person's relationship. It understands that some people simply grow out of substance misuse while others get into trouble. It understands change in a completely different way than previous models have. And it starts from a foundation of realism and compassion.

Harm reduction seeks to understand *why* each person develops a relationship with drugs. At least half of the people who have emotional and mental health problems also have problems with drugs, vastly more than the general population. Since most drugs are virtually the same as, and some *are,* prescription drugs, we subscribe to the self-medication hypothesis of drug use. Just because the drugs cause or exacerbate some problems doesn't mean they are not also a solution to others. Drugs interact in unique ways with each individual's physical, mental, emotional, and spiritual life and there is no single explanation for what most people call

> The fact that substances can cause problems doesn't mean they haven't helped solve others.

"addiction." Instead, harm reduction helps each person define his or her own particular problems related to drug use.

Harm reduction means being free—free of punitive sanctions for what you choose to put into your body and free of the fear, stigma, and shame that accompany your choice to use drugs.

Harm reduction is *not,* however, an easy way out. It's not an "excuse" to ignore the harm your use might be causing. Harm reduction is, in fact, very hard work. Most of us don't quit unhealthy habits and start healthy ones just because someone says so or just because it's the "right" thing to do. But that doesn't mean we do nothing at all. Harm reduction offers strategies and tools that help people manage or change their relationships with drugs without the need to go from 0 to 60. Or from 60 to 0.

Change doesn't happen overnight. But in America we like to think it does. Although it originated as part of an ad campaign, "just do it" has become a powerful meme that tells us not to waste time *thinking* about a problem or challenge but to get out there and *do* something about it. In our current culture of prohibition, *doing* means *quitting.* But how on earth do we know whether we want to quit when we haven't even analyzed the problem? Unfortunately, if we say *"No!"* we are labeled "unmotivated." Most of us do not lack *motivation* to change—we are more often *ambivalent,* of two minds, torn between the devil we know and the devil we don't. Change is scary. We don't know who we will be and whether we can handle the responsibilities of a different life. Harm reduction understands and embraces ambivalence. Having mixed feelings is actually healthy: it means you're able to see the pros, the cons, and the gray areas in between.

No one would suggest that you leave your husband or wife of 10, 20, or 30 years as soon as you get that "Oh, no, what have I been doing?" feeling. That sudden thud of reality that your relationship is a mess, even if the two of you have been fighting since the day you married, doesn't mean you're packing your bags tonight. You talk, you fight some more, you wonder how the kids would handle a divorce, you try to imagine yourself single again, and you just can't see it. The same is true for relationships with drugs. Realizing you have a problem takes time, as does figuring out whether you want to do something about it. And if drugs are helping you cope with something else equally or more serious, the process is even more complicated.

But, normal as it is, ambivalence can be paralyzing. Take heart. Being stuck on the fence is a reasonable reaction to the sinking feeling that you're going to be pressured to *do* something. Teetering on the fence is the legitimate beginning of the process of change. You don't have to *do* anything.

You can think without having to decide. You can even try different things without committing. No pressure.

A Different Language

You might have noticed already our use of different terminology than you are accustomed to hearing. Harm reduction has both embraced and created

> The language of harm reduction reflects the full range of drug experiences and options for change.

a language that reflects the full range of experiences with drugs and allows for the full range of options for change. It is a language grounded in research, a precise language that allows us to accurately understand each person's relationship with drugs and to select realistic options for change.

- *Substance (or drug) use and misuse*: We use these terms rather than *addiction*. Addiction is not actually a medical term, and is nowhere in the U.S. or European diagnostic manuals of medical and mental health disorders. The term is used too often and too casually to refer to *any* excessive behavior that we don't like in ourselves or others, rendering the word virtually meaningless as well as insulting to people who have *real* problems with drugs or compulsive behaviors. And the words *addict* and *alcoholic* carry an enormous amount of stigma in our society, stigma that negatively affects the person suffering as well as those who love him or her. We find the terms substance *use* and substance *misuse* more accurate. The former recognizes that the vast majority of Americans use alcohol and other drugs without issue. The latter is a neutral word that means using a substance in ways other than you intended.

- *Relationship with drugs*: Calling one's drug use a relationship highlights the emotional connections that people develop with the drugs they use. This term also shows respect for people who are struggling to balance the positive and negative results of their use.

- *Continuum of drug use*: Substance use occurs on a *continuum* that ranges from no use at all to harmless use to chaotic, out-of-control use, the kind that is often thought of as "addiction." In other words, people have different *levels* or *patterns* of use. Even for people whose substance use is harmful, their relationship with drugs can be healthy at other times; see the next page for revealing statistics (in the box). Each person's pattern is different, and each person can change in many directions. People also can have problems with some drugs and not others. We have seen people over the last 30 years who have problematic relationships with alcohol but not with marijuana, or who get in trouble with speed but drink moderately, including after they quit using speed. We have worked with people whose use is chaotic, then they learn to moderate, yet they still have the occasional binge. We have also worked with many people whose goal is abstinence from all psychoactive substances, and they achieve that and happily move on.

• *Harm*: we use this term to refer to the negative consequences that can occur at *any* level of use. When we use the word *harm,* we have to be specific about exactly what harms each drug and each pattern are causing you and others in your life. It requires that we be precise, and that precision helps us to prioritize things that need to change.

> Harms can occur at any point and should be addressed, regardless of whether a person is "addicted."

- Of the 70% of Americans who *use* alcohol in any given year, 6.6% have problems. And 90% of *heavy* drinkers are not "alcoholic" (word used in the study).

- Of the 9.4% of Americans 12 and over who *use* illegal drugs, 2.6% *misuse* them.

- Rates of substance misuse decline steadily over the lifespan. Many people (estimates vary) who *do* progress to one of the more serious levels of use back off on their own, without any help.

- Whereas 3.5% of adolescents and 7.5% of young adults misuse illegal drugs, 3.1% of adults between the ages of 26 and 44 do so, and only 1.1% of adults over 45, diminishing to almost 0 after 65. Likewise, rates of alcohol misuse slow over time from 13% for young adults to 9.1%, then 5% down to 2.4% over the lifespan.

- In other words, research shows that most people slow down or quit (called maturing out) by the time they are in their 30s. Others go back and forth between heavy and moderate use or abstinence.

Data drawn from large-scale annual surveys conducted by the Substance Abuse and Mental Health Services Administration (SAMHSA) in addition to other studies on remission rates for substance use disorders. See the Resources for a listing of data sources.

And a Different Practice . . .

Harm reduction is not about "getting clean":

> Unlike traditional "quit now and forever" programs, it is not about stopping all use of drugs, unless that is your goal.

> It is not about quitting drugs or alcohol in the hope that simply not having these things in your body will solve all your problems.

> It is not about determining, once and for all, whether you are an "addict."

> It is not based on an all-or-nothing attitude: drink *or* be on the wagon, use *or* quit, be clean *or* dirty, and so on.

Harm reduction invites you to address both your substance use *and* the issues that lie behind it. It asks you to recognize the harmful impacts—on you, your family, and your community—of your substance use, and it asks you to understand yourself and what drives your relationship with drugs. It challenges you to address the issues facing you, clearly and honestly, and it asks you to reduce harm. Whether or not you need to quit, it *does* mean you probably need to change *something*.

We appreciate the magnitude of such a challenge. If most of us had to strip down and look at our lives with brutal honesty, we'd climb into the nearest dark hole with as much of our drug of choice as money could buy and stay there till hell froze over. To some degree, we all avoid looking closely at the damage, pain, anger, sadness, loneliness, or depression in our lives. And we do so for an understandable reason: it hurts to live it, and it hurts to think about it.

Practicing harm reduction means taking an active interest in your own welfare and the welfare of those around you. It means being curious about why you drink or use. It means reviewing how you got here, why you started using in the first place, and how you got to the point of needing this book. It means examining, *without harsh judgments,* the risks of your drinking and the trouble you've gotten into because of it. It means accepting, *without guilt,* that you like things about your drugs, that they are helpful or pleasurable, even if they cause problems. Finally, it means reducing harm, and for each of you that will mean something different.

> Circular as it sounds, the goal of harm reduction is the reduction of harm.

What does this look like? Maybe you begin by making sure you always have a ride home from the bar so you're not driving drunk. Then you quit drinking gin and stick with beer because the piercing headache that accompanies your gin hangover makes you argumentative at work. Then you drink less beer. You realize you've been depressed for a while, and you start taking antidepressant medication. Maybe you find a therapist who knows about harm reduction and doesn't say you have to quit before you can talk about your problems. Maybe you stop smoking pot for a while so that you can study and pass your exams. You exercise. You eat before you drink. You talk to a friend who also uses meth, and together you agree to party no more than once a month, to quit by noon on Sunday, and to always have condoms in your pocket.

If, for you, reducing harm means abstaining entirely, that's fine. But if it means beginning with tiny changes that move you in a positive direction, that's fine too. If it means drinking, but for the first time in your life not driving drunk, that's wonderful. If it means limiting your marijuana use to evenings before dinner or only after the kids are in bed, then you have made a mature and healthy choice. If it means getting more sleep on Sunday so you don't need a hit of speed to get through Monday, you're on your way. That's the reality of change for most of us. We do as much as we can the best way we can. And that's harm reduction.

. . . With a Lot of History behind It

In the "addictions" field, harm reduction is a new approach. Although it's been known by that name since the early 1980s, it's still new to most individuals and still resisted by conventional treatment systems that subscribe to the idea that total abstinence is the only way to resolve problems with drugs.

On the other hand, harm reduction is not new at all; most of us practice it without even thinking. Harm reduction is wearing seat belts or motorcycle helmets. So is not drinking and driving—we do not forbid either somewhat risky activity; what we avoid is doing them at the same time. Preventive medicine—vaccinations, breast exams, prenatal care, and regular check-ups—is harm reduction; it lowers the *risk* of contracting diseases and having other health problems. Harm reduction is deciding it's time to start going to sleep before midnight. It is wearing sunglasses after years of squinting at the lake or on the ski slopes. In other words, harm reduction is just good common sense combined with some awareness of risk.

We are pretty sure that you have practiced harm reduction with at least some of your drugs. You might have cut down or quit for family holidays, funerals, a child's graduation, or important work projects, then resumed your usual habits. You might have quit for periods of time (a drug holiday) to rest, lose weight, or sat-

> We all practice harm reduction—it's just a combination of common sense and awareness of risk.

isfy a partner. You might have switched from spirits to beer, from alcohol to marijuana, or from shooting to smoking heroin. Even if you have not done these things yet, you have come to this book, so you are thinking about it.

> The reality of change: We do as much as we can the best way we can.

Finally, people change their substance use all the time. Most young people who have drunk alcohol and used drugs heavily reduce their use to nonharmful levels by the time they are 30. Most people who drink do so responsibly. That is true of drug users too, it is just not widely known because our national hysteria about illegal drug use keeps the ways that drug users manage their use underground. Each drug has a natural history and an expiration date, each slightly different, a natural course that waxes and then wanes over a period of years. If you think about the history of your own drug use, you will probably find that this is true for you too, for some of your drugs if not all.

. . . And Supported by a Great Deal of Evidence

Harm reduction offers a wide menu of options for changing your relationship with drugs without necessarily quitting. Its interventions come from decades of well-researched models and interventions in public health, medicine, and psychology. How does this work? Among many evidence-supported harm reduction strategies and interventions are:

Public Health Strategies

- *Needle exchange programs*: In communities where they operate, the rates of HIV and other blood-borne diseases are much lower than in communities where sterile syringes are unavailable, according to thousands of studies.

- *Naloxone*: The overdose reversal medication saves lives—10,000 between 1996 and 2010, according to the Centers for Disease Control.

- *Supervised injection facilities (SIFs)*: Hygienic facilities staffed by medical and support staff reduce disease transmission, prevent overdose, and provide access to drug treatment and other health care.

- *Ignition interlock systems*: These mechanisms, which prevent a car from starting if a person is under the influence of alcohol, prevent drinking and driving.

Addiction Medicine and Psychiatry

- *Opioid substitution therapy (OST)*: Methadone and buprenorphine are the most effective treatment for opioid misuse, especially when combined with other health, mental health, and socioeconomic support. OST lowers "street" drug use and crime and improves health and employment.

- *Alcohol craving medicines*: These evolve with research. Currently naltrexone is the medicine showing greatest efficacy in lowering alcohol craving.

- *Psychiatric medication*: Accurate diagnosis and treatment for conditions that people are self-medicating, such as attention-deficit/hyperactivity disorder (ADHD), depression, and anxiety, help people to manage their "street" drug use.

Behavior Change and Psychological Models

- *Moderation or controlled drinking*: 50% of people who have had alcohol problems drink "asymptomatically." There are various moderate drinking methods that help to achieve this, such as Moderation Management (*www.moderatedrinking.com, www.moderation.org*), HAMS (Harm Reduction, Abstinence, and Moderation Support, *www.hamsnetwork.org*), Guided Self-Change (*www.nova.edu/gsc/index.html*), CheckUp and Choices (*www.checkupandchoices.com*), and the method outlined in the National Institute of Alcoholism and Alcohol Abuse "Rethinking Drinking" pamphlet (*www.rethinkingdrinking.niaaa.nih.gov*).

- *Multipronged approaches*: Problems with substances result from an interaction between the drugs, the person, and his or her environment. This research-based model, developed by a psychiatrist who was studying heroin and cocaine users in the 1970s, is a foundation of harm reduction. Identifying and prioritizing issues in any of these three realms is more effective than always assuming that we must start by tackling the drugs. For example, using heroin alone increases the risk of a fatal overdose. Simply using with someone else ensures life-saving intervention and increases the likelihood that eventually you will reduce your use or quit.

- *Realistic change*: Evidence shows that people progress through different stages of change, each of which requires a different kind of focus and effort. Action, just doing it, is not where everyone is, even after they accept they have a problem. In the words of Alex Wodak, Australian physician and harm reduction pioneer, "80% of something is better than 100% of nothing."

- *Self-determination*: Individual choice is highly correlated with motivation, health, and a sense of well-being. Coercion, on the other hand, is correlated with low motivation and poor outcomes.

- *Relationships*: Being in contact with people who support rather than punish promotes motivation.

- *Empathy*: Deep understanding from others helps to mobilize motivation and is the foundation of a supportive relationship. *And empathy means understanding you from your point of view.*

- *Psychotherapy*: Therapy is as effective as other treatment interventions and is important for people who have complicating emotional or major mental health issues.

Socioeconomic Support

For people who have lost everything—family, income, housing, a clean criminal record, and health—survival is a constant source of stress. Providing services and support without barriers is essential to their ability to regain some stability. Housing First initiatives, job readiness training and placement, reentry programs, benefits advocacy, and primary care services are essential to the overall well-being of people who are marginalized. They are integral to harm reduction. Because people who are marginalized are much more likely to develop problematic drug use and mental health issues, respectful treatments are also essential to their ability to recover and take their place in society.

Integration of Many Different Strategies

Harm reduction integrates many different interventions—public health, medical, counseling, and practical—and customizes interventions to each individual. Harm reduction is flexible, offers a menu of options for change, and believes in whatever works to reduce harm and improve health. These things are key to its effectiveness, as found in a 2010 international review of the efficacy of harm reduction (*www.drugpolicy.org/resource/harm-reduction-evidence-impacts-and-challenges*).

What Harm Reduction Offers

Unconditional Welcome

Come as you are is the mantra of harm reduction—anyone is welcome, regardless of his or her relationship with drugs, goals for future use, and motivation to change. Any route to change is supported, and every positive change applauded. Start where you are, not where you or someone else thinks you should be, and trust your gut when it says, "That isn't going to work for me" or "That sounds like a great idea." You'll stand a better chance of making a plan that will work for *you*.

Respect

Many people will tell you that if you follow your own wisdom, you're trying to do it "your way"—followed quickly by "Your 'stinking thinking' got you into this mess in the first place." And "It works if you work it." Your only option then is to surrender and follow "the program," without regard for whether the program (almost always based on the 12 steps) is right for *you*.

Harm reduction understand that all kinds of people use all sorts of drugs, and there is nothing inherently wrong with this. Even at the worst of times, people retain their humanity and their self-knowledge. We have never met a drug misuser who had no awareness of at least some of the harms he or she was incurring. Treating a person with dignity and respect opens the door for a real conversation to occur.

Harm reduction treats *you* as the expert. Only you know your pain. Only you can evaluate what you need and why you use drugs to fill that need. Only you know whether you can quit heroin, alcohol, *and* cigarettes, *or not*. Harm reduction trusts that, consciously or not, you are always balancing the risks and benefits of using versus quitting or cutting down. Our job is to help you find more options between keeping on as you are and quitting altogether.

Curiosity

Harm reduction is *interested* in your relationship with drugs. Many people change things all the time without thinking much about them. But for people who are really attached to their drinking and their drugs, it is important to understand *what* you are attached to and what you would be giving up if you changed. What does it mean to you? Is it medicine? Is it how you feel about yourself? In harm reduction, we ask dozens of questions. **And we do so completely without judgment.**

Safety before All Else (Do Less Harm)

Before anything else, harm reduction pays attention to safety—both yours and others'. Safety means reducing the *harm* of your drug use without necessarily reducing how *much* you use. Not drinking and driving, sterile syringes and safe crack pipes, taking care of the kids, and loading up on condoms when you set out for a party are but a few of the harm-reducing possibilities that harm reductionists keep foremost in our minds. Safer use strategies can be implemented by changing the route of administration (for example, switching from shooting to inhaling, from smoking to eating) or adjusting the frequency, the timing, or the amount of one's use. Easier said than done when you are burdened with trouble or feeling reluctant, but we help you explore safety options as quickly as possible. The bottom line is: **You don't have to quit to be safe!** We believe that drug users have as much right to be safe and healthy as anyone else. People say, "You have to bottom out before you'll be ready to *do* something." To that we say, "Bottoming out kills."

Real Information: "Just Say Know" Instead of "Just Say No"

Harm reduction offers accurate and unbiased information about drugs. And it offers this information to *everyone* who uses, not just those who have been identified as "addicts." After all, people might not *know* that you can overdose the first time you try heroin, or that what seems like a drinking game can become lethal, or that you need to drink lots of water if you're using ecstasy and dancing to avoid dangerously overheating. "Just Say No" messages deprive people of real and detailed information that saves lives.

Harm reduction assumes that people are intelligent and capable of making informed choices *if they have the information they need* (see the box on the next page).

- **Know** what and how much you are using—the potency as well as the amount.

- **Know** why you are using—what you are looking for in each dose, what you expect to happen, and what your vulnerabilities are.

- **Know** your surroundings—the place and the people—and the extent to which they are safe and supportive or might put you at risk of harm.

- **Know** your limits—the line between just enough and too much, FOR YOU.

Tips to Care for Yourself While You're Using

Harm reduction means taking care of yourself, regardless of the status of your drug use. Eat, drink water, breathe fresh air. Get your emotional and mental health needs attended to, formally or informally. Get prenatal care without fear of criminal sanctions. (Check the laws of the state you live in to find out if there are penalties for pregnant women who use drugs.) Spend at least a little time around people who care about you and treat you kindly. Treat yourself kindly. Stay away from judgment, rejection, and dogma. Some of these things require the cooperation of therapists, doctors, and state laws. Others you can do by yourself or with the help of friends.

Any Positive Change

Harm reduction values *any* movement in the direction of greater health and well-being, however small. Changing the time of day—just starting a couple of hours later so you can eat a big breakfast—taking a break, drinking a couple of pints of water, or taking a nap can be of huge benefit to your health. Some people moderate their use of all drugs, while others abstain from all; some abstain from some and moderate others, while still others abstain or moderate most of the time and then enjoy the occasional episode of intoxication. **We in the harm reduction community believe that "absence of problematic substance use," alongside a sense of well-being, optimal health, and satisfaction with life, defines being fully out of harm's way. What others call "recovery" we call being *over it*.**

> Being *over it* means having a sense of well-being, optimal health, satisfaction with life, and a nonproblematic relationship with drugs.

Self-Efficacy

"Success breeds success." We believe in this old adage. And there is plenty of research to back it up. Self-efficacy is the belief that "I can." It is having the confidence in your ability to accomplish a specific task or goal. Self-efficacy is an important concept in the field of psychology, and it is one of the single greatest determinants of motivation and success. In other words, belief in yourself predicts success. Belief in failure, on the other hand . . . well, you get the point. It's called the "What the hell?" syndrome. What this leads us to conclude is that it is better to make small changes that you can count on than to aim for goals that are too large to meet in a meaningful time frame.

Could Harm Reduction Be for You?

Everyone can benefit from harm reduction, whether you identify as a problematic drug user, you overindulge in other things that you would like to change, or you simply like its philosophy and practices as a way of approaching any problem.

> You are the only one with the power to choose what's best for you.

What If You Don't Want to Acknowledge Harm?

By now you've probably been told that your unwillingness to quit or even to acknowledge the harmful consequences of your habit means you're "in denial." Besides the likelihood that you are ambivalent about doing something different, or you still aren't convinced of what the problem is, looking at harm is *painful,* especially if the damage is serious. Your head hurts, your stomach churns, you feel hopeless, you hate yourself and your life, and that dark hole looks awfully tempting. These are some of the very things that *drive* drinking and using.

> "I feel guilty about how much money I've blown on crack, so I smoke more to erase the guilt."

> "I'm already a junkie with AIDS, so why bother using clean needles?"

> "My wife left because I drink, so what the hell? Might as well keep drinking."

- **Harm reduction is for *anyone* who has developed problems with alcohol or other drugs.** You don't have to define yourself (or let someone else define you) as an "addict" or an "alcoholic." You don't have to "hit bottom" before you can get better. You don't have to be living on the street, getting arrested, courting disaster, alienating everyone, or living in chaos before you recognize the need to do something different.

- **It's for you if your life as a party animal is starting to catch up to you**—if your social use of alcohol or other drugs has become more pervasive and is affecting your work, your relationships, and your finances.

- **It's for you if you feel like you're just not at your best these days and you wonder how in the world you got to this point**—where you're drinking every single evening, and no longer a glass of wine or two with dinner but a couple of martinis followed by a bottle of wine. Or you've smoked just a little pot for all of your adult life and all of a sudden feel like your life hasn't changed in 20 years.

- **Harm reduction is for people who have co-occurring emotional problems or complicating medical issues.**

- **It's for you if you like to solve problems your own way but still want a science-based method.**

- **Harm reduction is for people who have tried the standard treatment and 12-step options and found them unsatisfactory.** Some people want to be in charge of their own lives and find the idea of powerlessness ridiculous. Others experience powerlessness as terrifying because it is the very real condition that they experience every day; why on earth would they *embrace* it? Still others want and need a more complex psychological approach that explores the reasons and the meaning behind their relationship with drugs.

- **Harm reduction is for those who have been denied therapy "until they *do* something about their drug problem," which usually means going to AA, NA, or drug treatment.** Some people want or need therapy for vital and life-saving reasons and can't even think about changing anything until they sort out the relationship between their drugs, their physical and emotional states, and their environment.

- **Harm reduction is also for people who have suffered treatment trauma.** By "treatment trauma" we mean experiences in treatment that have *caused* harm—experiences such as confrontation, verbal abuse, demeaning language, exclusion or isolation from the group, and sometimes outright brutality.

- **Harm reduction is for people who don't want to be abstinent to solve their problems with drugs.** Harm reduction embraces many avenues of change and has strategies to accomplish them. The three broad directions that people choose are safer use, moderation, and abstinence. (Yes, it is a myth that harm reduction is opposed to abstinence.) All are very well-founded and successful routes to change and health.

- **And finally, harm reduction is for people who want to be no longer under the influence of either drugs or addiction dogma, who want to get over it once and for all.**

Don't freak out! This reaction is normal. Looking at harm is a big step, and a very painful one if the damage is serious. Take a break. Take your time. Give this book to your cousin who *really* needs it. Or just leave it on the shelf and head for the bar. (Just don't drive to get there!) When you're ready, when you become curious or more relaxed, when some other crisis in your life has calmed down, when you feel it's safe to move forward, or when you can't stand the pain anymore, you can start again. Wait until you *want* to pick up the book. In the meantime, skip to Chapter 9 to get more tips on how to take care of yourself while still using. Or go straight to Chapter 11, where we discuss how to find help that will honor your self-determination and help you change at your pace.

It's YOUR life.

It works best if you define your problems.

Change is most successful if you choose a path that YOU can follow.

2 Why Do People Use Drugs?

> *The ubiquity of drug use is so striking that it must represent a basic human appetite.*
> —ANDREW WEIL, an early pioneer in the field of ethnobotany of medicinal plants, now better known as an advocate of holistic medicine

People use drugs. We get drunk, we get high, we seek heightened or altered states of consciousness, we are curious. We have been brewing beer for thousands of years. We have been selecting medicinal herbs and hallucinogenic plants for the same thousands of years. We have dedicated enormous effort to cultivating teas and coffee beans. We humans have been taking drugs to celebrate victories and meaningful occasions, to relieve stress and illness, to have fun, and to enhance religious rituals since we first walked on this planet. And most of us still do. (So do animals!) Our brains have all the equipment in place to seek pleasure and relieve pain. Dopamine and endorphins and norepinephrine and anandamide—these are all natural substances in the brain (neurotransmitters, aka brain chemicals) responsible for feelings of pleasure, soothing, pain relief, alertness, and bliss.

All drugs either mimic or stimulate these and a few other brain chemicals, thereby enhancing processes that are already part of normal brain functioning. And it is not just drugs that give us pleasure, lubricate social interactions, achieve states of ecstasy, alter or heighten perception, relieve pain, soothe discomfort, sharpen focus, and enhance performance. So do stunning landscapes, massage, yoga poses, cardio exercise, extreme sports, a perfectly cooked meal, great sex, or twirling around in circles until you fall down.

Unfortunately, the good that drugs, including alcohol, do is kept hush-hush because asserting any positive impact breaks a taboo that has existed in America for more than 200 years. Getting out of one's mind, being pain free, or experiencing pleasure for pleasure's sake flies in the face of the dominant Puritan ethic of colonial America that insists that hard work and struggle are the keys to progress, success, and salvation. "No pain, no gain!" To this day, ecstasy (the feeling, not the drug!) and other extreme mind states make us nervous that we are not attending to our economic, social, and moral responsibilities. So we use in secret, or we sheepishly admit to the hangover we got after the fabulous party we enjoyed the night before.

This was not always true. Most cultures had important rituals that involved states of ecstasy or psychic journeys, often made possible by drugs. In the United States, however, we became divorced from our roots. Native Americans used tobacco and peyote. Colonists drank much more alcohol per person than we do today. Both of those uses were embedded in cultural rituals, whether religion or the sharing of a meal in a tavern. There were few problems. With the advent of the Revolutionary War, the Industrial Revolution, and the westward expansion, public drunkenness emerged and, along with it, a crusade to stamp out all use of alcohol.

This *moral model* is the earliest way of understanding the U.S. response to intoxication. Early-19th-century Americans decided that those who over-imbibe are suffering from a moral weakness of character. Temperance movements that began in the early 19th century evolved into a full-scale war on drugs in the 20th, eventually leading to total prohibition—of alcohol for 13 years and of most other intoxicating drugs since 1914. Today, two centuries later, the moralistic judgments that stem from prohibition remain in the minds of Americans. We now risk stigma, discrimination, punitive sanctions, and jail if we are caught using (most) drugs. Most of us drink, but we rarely brag about getting *drunk.* And when people hear the phrase *using drugs,* there is an automatic association with crime, antisocial behavior, dirt, skid row, poverty, laziness, and other "bad" things. Employers, schools, and sports teams test for drugs. Cops arrest and jail people, and judges sentence people. Then, once convicted of a drug felony, we are denied student loans (a surefire way to keep people from pulling themselves out of a life of using drugs) and the right to vote, a fundamental right of citizenship. *No wonder we don't want to talk about drugs or drug use!*

But **people use drugs for reasons**, as we explained in the first chapter. And drugs, including alcohol, are more closely associated with relief, fun, relaxation, altered perception, higher states of consciousness, and pleasure than they are with crime, antisocial behavior, and the like. (Of course, the Puritan work ethic also decries too much pleasure of any kind, so drugs just can't win.) Still, we insist on coming down harder on those who ease pain and stress with drugs or alcohol than on those who use cookies or action movies to comfort or distract themselves. We draw a sharp

> Let's be cautious about taking away what helps, even if it also causes harm, before understanding the help it provides.

distinction between self-administered substances and prescription drugs. We focus on the harm of substance use to the exclusion of the benefits. All of these attitudes perpetuate some muddles addressed in the box on page 27.

So Why *Do* People Use Drugs?

According to neuropsychologist Allan Schore, among others, we are all wired to seek pleasure and avoid pain, and in a general sense that's what all drugs help us do. Anthropologists and cultural historians add that, throughout human history, a desire to alter consciousness has also been a driving force. Psychopharmacologist Ronald Siegel, best known now for his work in mindfulness, did much research in both human and animal desires to get high and believes that it is a universal desire. Later in the chapter, we offer brief descriptions of the benefits of each type of drug, but the broader reasons for using drugs typically fall into the following categories.

> People use drugs for reasons—reasons that need to be understood, not criticized and suppressed.

Intoxication

Around the world throughout history, drugs have been used in rituals with the goal of exploring the self, communing with the physical world, exploring the mysteries of the spirit world, and expanding consciousness beyond the everyday business of life. With the exception of the Inuit (who had no access to plants and therefore no drugs until alcohol was introduced to them) there is no established society in the history of the world that has *not* used psychoactive drugs. The study of the use of psychoactive drugs is called *intoxicology*. It arose around the time that cultural historians became interested in the nutritional and gastronomic habits of human societies. It was at this time, in 1973, that Andrew Weil uttered the statement that we quote at the beginning of the chapter. Weil pointed out that children spinning in circles until they are so dizzy they fall down is little different from a teenager's attempts to get drunk or an adult's pursuit of psychedelic experiences. Michael Pollan, before he became famous as a food historian and nutritional adviser, explored the strange dichotomy between prescribed medicines and self-grown and self-prescribed drugs. In his

> To get drunk, to get high, to get out of one's mind has been a natural phenomenon throughout human history.

Clearing Up Some Muddles

The "Drug" Label

At least in part because they are illegal, "drugs" are merged into one potent threat that lives underground and drags innocent young people into a life of corruption and criminality. We do not think with any precision about what these substances actually *are,* or about the unique uses, history, and culture of each individual substance. Because we have decided to make drugs illegal, we cannot study them, their effects, or their benefits and harms dispassionately and in detail. Because it is legal, an exception is made for alcohol. We refine and revere "craft" beers, "fine" wines, and "artisanal" whiskeys and read weekly columns and hundreds of books dedicated to mixology, the art and science of the cocktail. We have also developed standards for moderate drinking that are endorsed by the U.S. National Institutes of Health.

Use Merges into Abuse

One thing that makes it difficult to understand why people *use* drugs is that we keep using terms like *abuse* and *addiction*. While we do a pretty good job of distinguishing between drinking and "alcoholism," we have a harder time doing this when we talk about drugs. Because they are illegal and therefore their use is *wrong,* drug use is deviant. Therefore, *all drug use is abuse*. Take a look at your local newspaper, listen to broadcasts about drugs, read almost any book or pamphlet, and you'll probably see what we mean. This is the climate in which we view drug use, and even though our attitudes are changing, this muddling of use/abuse is still pervasive.

Abuse = Addiction = Disease

If all use is abuse, then by extension all drug users are addicts, since addiction is how we label problematic substance use. For example, we almost never hear anyone outside of the harm reduction community refer to a heroin "user." It seems that the words *heroin* and *addict* are joined at the hip. And yet only 23% of people who use heroin, for example, become "addicted," according to the National Institute on Drug Abuse. Since addiction is supposedly a disease, all drug users are therefore diseased. Such assumptions and oversimplifications make it difficult to look at why most people use alcohol or drugs and why only some of them get in trouble (the subject of Chapter 4).

book *Botany of Desire,* he discusses the close affinity between people and psychoactive plants, marijuana in particular. He concludes that it is an interdependent relationship that has existed for millennia.

Cultural and Religious Ritual

Prior to the Industrial Revolution in the West, much intoxication occurred in the context of religious and spiritual ritual. From the alcohol-infused bacchanalia to the ritual of the Eleusinian mysteries (suspected to involve psychedelics), ayahuasca and peyote ceremonies, and the sacrament of ganja in the Rastafarian religion to the incorporation of wine into Christian sacrament, many drugs have been used to enhance spiritual enlightenment. In secular societies where religion is not the focal point of gathering and celebrating, social rituals have taken their place.

Recreation/Pleasure

While ritual religious or ceremonial use is still common in many cultures, with the secularization of many societies, recreational use has become the norm in many places. Sometimes it's entirely nonceremonial (relaxing with a cocktail after work), and other times it's integral to communal events and ceremonies—champagne at a wedding, beer at baseball games, marijuana at a music event, speed or cocaine at a party. Ecstatic drug experiences—ecstasy at raves, LSD and other hallucinogens, ketamine, even drunken fraternity parties—continue to thrive, with more or less awareness about the power of the drugs and the mind-altering potential of the experiences. The spiritual or religious associations have been lost in most of these cases, but the drug experiences are much the same as thousands of years ago. The big difference is that drug-induced experiences, with the exception of those lubricated by alcohol, are not embraced as a part of mainstream society in the United States.

Diet

Up through colonial America, beer resembled a food more than a recreational alcoholic beverage. Thick, full of nutrients from grains, and often cleaner than the available water, it provided sustenance to people whose diets were simple. Coca leaf has been essential to maintaining stamina for people who work hard at high altitudes in the Andes. Mormon tea became a staple in early Mormon Utah. It contains the drug ephedrine, which offers a comparable stimulation to a culture that bans all drugs including caffeine. While wine might not be classed a food, most people in Mediterranean cultures would not think of excluding it from meals. Does it supply essential nutrients? Maybe, maybe not. Is a meal complete without it? *No.*

Medicine

Medicinal use of marijuana shows up in 5,000-year-old Chinese medical texts. Poppy seeds, some still nestled in pipes, have been found in millennia-old graves all over Europe. All drugs were either discovered (opium and marijuana), derived from natural substances (morphine), chemically modified from a natural substance (heroin and methamphetamine), or manufactured (ecstasy) to treat a wide variety of physical ailments, from excruciating pain to arthritis to glaucoma to asthma. Drugs also relieve emotional pain and discomfort. Upper-class 19th-century women found that the opioids prescribed for menstrual cramps also soothed their social anxiety or relieved their boredom, just as 1950s housewives discovered the benefits of barbiturates. Many people with schizophrenia find that alcohol and nicotine relieve psychotic symptoms (and they smoke at three times the rate of the general population); as we mentioned in Chapter 1, there is a strong correlation between childhood trauma and adult substance misuse; and alcohol has helped many a shy person overcome social anxiety.

Coping

We manage the stress of life in a variety of ways. As teenagers we hit an age of awkwardness and self-consciousness. Unless we were supremely successful socially, academically, or athletically, or we lived in an easygoing and supportive community, this was at least a slightly painful period of life. Some of us had great mentors. Some joined the church choir or formed a band. Some of us got into extreme sports. Some became rebels and joined protest movements. Some of us buried ourselves in books. And some found drugs. Some of us were multitalented multitaskers and did it all! Whatever we found, any and all of those pursuits are normal parts of existence, including the drugs.

Choice

We make choices to use drugs for many reasons: social pressure, excitement and curiosity, a wish to escape something unpleasant, a desire to see the world differently—more clearly or more fuzzily—or just because they are there. Some drug use is intentional and planned, other use less so. If you think about your own early drug experiences, you will remember the reasons that you picked up your first drink, smoked your first cigarette or joint, snorted your first speed, shot your first heroin, or popped your first pill. Sometimes our choice of drug is controlled and constrained by its availability and its cost. If it's not around or we can't afford to buy it, chances are we won't be using it. At least not often enough to develop a habit! We also make choices based on what we refer to as context. Some drugs combine better with certain activities than others. You don't generally take a stimulant if you want to have a mellow conversation with a new lover. You might, however, smoke some weed. If you are socially awkward and going to a party, you might want to get lubricated with alcohol first. If the smell of alcohol on your breath seems like a bad idea, an Ativan will do the trick, too.

Bruce Alexander, who has spent a professional lifetime studying and understanding "addictive" behavior, thinks of drug use as a choice in the absence of other options. This was made apparent in his Rat Park study where rats that were housed in an environment similar to a rat's natural living environment used far less morphine than rats who were isolated in typical laboratory cages.

> Drug use is often chosen when it seems there are no other options.

The Social Influences on Choice

We are social creatures, and our choice of drugs is often determined to some extent by our culture and our wish to belong.

Belonging and Not Belonging

Drugs are among the many lubricants used to enhance social relationships, creating a sense of community and bonding among people who use. It's not just belonging that might encourage drug use, however, but *not* belonging. A disproportionate number of gay, lesbian, bisexual, transgender, and queer people, and those questioning their sexuality or gender identity, use alcohol and other drugs. The assumption is that being a part of a stigmatized, and often bullied, group causes such fear and shame that the only way to cope sometimes is to get high. Many a gay person lived in terror through middle and high school, only to discover the relieving and euphoric qualities of alcohol, pot, or pills.

But you don't have to be part of a stigmatized group to feel pressure or discomfort. Am I smart enough, thin enough, beautiful or handsome enough, fit enough, rich enough, powerful enough? Do I live in the right neighborhood, in the right house? Am I hip enough? Do I listen to the right music, see the right films, wear the right clothes? Inadequacy in the face of pressure to conform to externally imposed standards is something we all face and is a demon that some have overcome through religion, therapy, or just plain age and maturity. Other people find drugs.

Social Networks

Social groupings, or networks, are often drug-specific. Some drugs are considered trendy and others bad. The debate between "junkies" and "crackheads" is a case in point—each group thinking the other is the lowest of the low. Alcohol swings both ways. Many cultures see alcohol as an important part of celebrations and rituals, or even just as an everyday part of a meal. They might see heroin use as the end of the line, the place of no hope. There are others, especially younger people, who think that alcohol is a sloppy drug, best used by older people, but that heroin is cool and, as long as it is clean and used properly, causes less bodily harm (they are right). The more you want to belong to a particular group, the harder it will be to say no to the heroin and drink the beer that you might actually prefer, or vice versa.

Sometimes choice doesn't even seem to be operating—it's just what you do! High school boys playing basketball, then hanging out smoking a blunt. Everyone in your group is doing it? Chances are you will too. College students going to a club or a game—if your friends tend to pregame/preparty (drink before even going out to drink more), you will too.

Last, but Not Least, Drugs Work!

People often choose the drug that fits best with their need or desire for pleasure, relief, or altered perception. Each class (type) of drug has its own chemical profile that targets specific neurotransmitters (brain chemicals) and creates effects that are unique to that drug. Those neurotransmitters, in turn, cause specific feeling states—euphoria and pleasure, excitement and arousal, relaxation and soothing, dreaminess, and sleep. In addition, most types of "recreational" drugs have accepted medical uses. For example, one might choose:

- Stimulants for ADHD
- Opioids for pain
- Marijuana for arthritis, multiple sclerosis, glaucoma, nausea, and the weight loss associated with AIDS or cancer.

Many "recreational" drugs are also chosen because of how they make us think, feel, or act differently:

- If you're feeling depressed, sluggish, bored, or plagued by low self-esteem, you might gravitate toward stimulants like amphetamines or cocaine.
- If you feel irritable, moody, or stressed, you might be drawn to opioids or marijuana.
- People who have experienced trauma might also find relief from the relaxing and memory-dulling effects of marijuana, the sedating effects of opioids or sedatives like Valium, or the relaxing and disinhibiting effects of alcohol. Or they might turn to dissociative anesthetics, which can give you an out-of-body experience and reduce self-consciousness. (Dissociation—when your mind separates itself from reality—just happens to be one of the main *protective* symptoms of posttraumatic stress.)

The quick reference at the back of the book gives a lot more detail about how drugs work. But for now, here are some highlights that indicate why people might choose certain drugs.

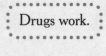

Drugs work.

Alcohol

Alcohol relaxes, stimulates, *and* disinhibits (loosens the tight rein you keep on yourself), so it's the drug of choice for people who feel shy, awkward, or anxious, especially socially anxious. Some people with schizophrenia have found that alcohol turns down the volume of their auditory hallucinations (voices).

Cannabis

Cannabis (marijuana) has an old and rich history around the world, with medicinal, relaxing, fun, and hallucinogenic properties. Some people experience pleasant feelings while others feel anxious or even paranoid. On the other hand, many people with anxiety feel calmed by it. With legalization, there are so many strains of cannabis now available with so many different medicinal and recreational effects that new information is coming out all the time.

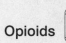

Opioids

Opioid drugs are the best medications in the world for pain relief. They also create a sense of euphoria and feelings of warmth and security. People with depression often find relief from the bleak outlook and emotional pain that are part of depression.

Stimulants

Stimulants, including caffeine, have been used for centuries for energy, alertness, and performance enhancement. Not to mention that speed and cocaine are great for sex (until they're not). The sense of expansiveness, energy, and powerfulness feels great for most anyone, especially people who are depressed or who feel emotionally flattened by their psychiatric medications.

Sedatives/Hypnotics

This class of drugs includes legal pharmaceuticals that are used to relieve anxiety, aid sleep, and generally provide relief from stress. Valium, Xanax, and Ambien are examples. They are excellent medicines when used properly, providing great relief with few negative side effects.

Nicotine

Nicotine increases activity in the areas of the brain responsible for concentration and focus—a useful effect for people with ADHD, for example. It also helps when you are anxious: 47% of people with serious mental illness use nicotine (as compared to 22% of people without).

Entheogens

Hallucinogens/psychedelics, ecstasy, and dissociative anesthetics are grouped under the larger category called *entheogens,* a term derived from the Greek that means "generating the divine within." All of these drugs have long histories of religious and other ceremonial uses.

Hallucinogenic or psychedelic drugs—among others, psilocybin mushrooms, peyote, LSD, marijuana sometimes, especially when it is eaten—create visual hallucinations, a sense of wonder and connection with the larger universe, and a capacity for introspection that is difficult to achieve outside of deep meditative states. Ongoing research is looking at whether they might be good treatments for both "addiction" to other drugs and posttraumatic stress disorder (PTSD).

Likewise, **ecstasy** is renowned for its ability to create feelings of well-being, warmth, love, and connection. Often called an *empathogen* for its ability to create emotional relatedness and empathy, it was used for many years as an aid in therapy, especially couple therapy, until it was banned in the 1980s. It, too, is enjoying renewed study as a treatment for PTSD.

Dissociative drugs produce a sense of wakeful dreaminess, precisely the purpose for which they were developed. Ketamine is particularly popular, but other dissociatives include PCP and nitrous oxide. In addition to being used as a party drug or a drug for spiritual journeys, ketamine is still used both in pediatric and veterinary medicine to sedate children or animals for surgical procedures when conscious sedation is necessary. (It has sometimes been referred to as a horse tranquilizer because of its use by veterinarians.)

Deliriants/Inhalants

Any drug can get you wasted—totally obliterated, out of your mind (delirious)—but some drugs really do it. Most drugs in this category are inhaled; thus their name. Inhalants include butyl and amyl nitrite, or poppers, used at parties and to enhance sexual encounters. Inhalants also include household and industrial solvents, glue, and gasoline. Why would people do this? Some people, like the kids who live parentless on the streets of cities like Nairobi, Karachi, or Rio, have no access to other drugs to help relieve the stress of trying to survive. Between 80 and 100% use inhalants. In South America, inhalants are the second most commonly used drug after marijuana among secondary-school students (most common in Brazil). Twenty percent of American and European kids use inhalants, many if not most of them poor and marginalized. Some kids get under the sink or stick their nose close to the gas pump because it's fascinating to feel the dizziness that comes with it (remember the twirling in circles?). For others, it's the only thing available and it's free. Finally, it's there to be done, it can be done under the radar, and kids are naturally curious.

Three People Who Are Struggling with Their Choices

Cheryl, Tyler, and Ruben use alcohol and other drugs for reasons such as those listed above. We'll follow them through the first half of the book so you can see how their relationships with drugs evolve.

Cheryl

Cheryl, 46, is an established and successful attorney. She has good friends in the Bay Area and a close relationship with her parents, who still live in the small Georgia town in which she was raised. She is on the board of a couple of local arts organizations and is quite respected in the community. She loves wine and often goes on wine-tasting trips with her friends. Her private grief is that she cannot seem to maintain long-term relationships with men. She dates, her relationships become intimate, but a few months after the sexual relationship has begun, the fighting starts. Conflicts seem to rage over everything, large and small. After many such relationships, it is clear that *she* is the common denominator.

As an African American woman raised in the small-town South in the not-enlightened-enough 1980s, the respect Cheryl has earned is a point of pride. She is ashamed that she has not completed her success by having a marriage and children. Cheryl doesn't argue with the fact that her drinking plays a part in escalating the conflicts in which she finds herself embroiled. Her dilemma is that she is too uptight to have sex without it. She craves sexual intimacy, but she is also afraid of it. What no one knows is that her oldest brother molested her for 3 years beginning when she was 8 years old. As is often the case, he told her he would kill her if she told anyone. The abuse stopped when he left home at 18. He was always difficult and is in and out of trouble now as an adult. Her parents have suffered so much over their oldest child that she could never bear to tell them about what he did to her. So it remained a secret until she sought therapy for her relationship problems.

Cheryl has another secret. A year ago she had some dental work and was given the opioid painkiller Vicodin. Never before, not even with a lot of alcohol, had she felt so calm and at ease. At first, after she didn't really need them anymore, she would just take one or two after work, sometimes with a little less alcohol than usual. But in the past few months she has started taking them every day and finds that if she doesn't, she gets irritable by the middle of the day. By the end of the day she is sweaty and anxious, so she gives in again, "just this once."

Cheryl is feeling less healthy, not eating well or exercising regularly, and not spending as much time with friends. Recently she was diagnosed with hypertension, and her doctor wants her to start taking medication. Everyone is focusing on the damage alcohol is doing to her health and her relationships. They don't know that she is actually drinking less because she is taking pills. They also don't know how much alcohol prevents her from having to notice her loneliness. Her friends have suggested that she go to Alcoholics Anonymous, but she gets mad at that advice. After all, she's not an alcoholic. She works, she has friends, and besides, she doesn't always drink too much. Plus, she's come a long way in her life and doesn't want to lose ground at this point in her life by being pigeonholed as an alcoholic. And she knows that she doesn't dare tell her friends about her pill use.

Tyler

Tyler, in his late 20s, enjoyed his reputation as a party animal. He could out-drink a sailor and use more speed than anyone else would dare. And yet, he not only managed to graduate from college, but has a great editorial job at a local newspaper that tolerates his occasional disappearances. He often starts his day with "just a bump" (of speed), but sometimes takes another one to get him through the afternoon. He routinely ends a workday by having a few drinks with friends at a local bar. He feels lonely sometimes, though, and has not had a serious relationship in his life. But he runs away from those feelings. His weekends are spent at clubs and at friends' houses, smoking meth and drinking rum and coke. (He started using speed during college to stay up late and study. Rum and coke was his first drink as a teenager; now it helps balance out the effects of meth.) He hooks up with women, but it never goes beyond a few times. Mondays are not a good day for him and, despite his youth, he is looking haggard.

Shortly after his 25th birthday, Tyler's best friend got married. At the bachelor party Tyler was surprised that it wasn't a drunken orgy, but rather a gathering of old friends who spent the evening telling tales of how stupid they and the groom were when they were younger. Of course Tyler had quite a few tales to tell. But the spirit of the evening was about growing up, putting away the wild times in favor of enjoying a mature relationship. Tyler made fun of his friend for giving up the good life, but the evening stuck with him.

Ruben

Ruben is a 31-year-old Latino gay man who works as a marketing specialist for a high-tech firm. He's been struggling lately, though. He had been HIV positive for years before being tested, and then delayed starting treatment because he felt so ashamed of being infected. Now that he was receiving treatment, though, his viral load wasn't going down as quickly as his doctor hoped and he was feeling a lot of fatigue. Complicating his illness is his pattern of drug use. Ruben refers to himself as a "garbage druggie," using pretty much anything that is around—cocaine, marijuana, ecstasy, poppers, alcohol, and "any little pretty pill."

Ruben had never had an easy life. Born a middle child among six children to migrant farm workers from Mexico, he was picked on, bullied, and attacked because from a young age it was clear that he was gay. He learned to hide his temper, avoid the biggest bullies, smoke a lot of marijuana, and surround himself with girls at school that he could entertain with his humor and feel some warmth from. His schoolwork suffered, and as he became an adult, he was unable to keep a job for any period of time. By the end of his 20s, though, he had turned things around and has now been employed steadily for 2 years.

He had long suffered from depression and anxiety as well as moodiness and paranoia that often caught others off guard. Then he moved to San Francisco. And his life changed overnight. For the first time he was popular and other men paid him a lot of attention. He could never establish an intimate relationship, though, settling for a series of sexual encounters fueled by alcohol and drugs. Even with all of the attention, he feels lonely a lot. Someday he hopes to settle down with the "perfect guy" and have children.

Each Drug Is Different, and Reasons Change over Time

Cheryl, Tyler, and Ruben are using different drugs for different reasons. And those reasons might have changed over time. It is important to consider why they started and why they keep on using. In some cases the reasons stay the same. In others they change.

Cheryl's Choices		
Drug	**Why I Started Using**	**Why I Use Now**
Wine	Social activity and enjoyment of good wine	Cope with loneliness and difficulty with relationships
Opioid pills	Postsurgical pain	Causes less irritability than alcohol; helps me reduce alcohol consumption

Tyler's Choices		
Drug	**Why I Started Using**	**Why I Use Now**
Meth (speed)	To stay up and study	To party and hook up with women
Rum and Coke	First drink I was given	It's still my favorite drink, and it helps mellow out the harsh effects of meth

Ruben's Choices		
Drug	**Why I Started Using**	**Why I Use Now**
Ecstasy	To dance and feel close to people	To look for a relationship
Alcohol	To calm my anxiety	It still helps with anxiety in social situations
Marijuana	Made me not care so much about being bullied	Helps me block out painful memories
Cocaine	Made me less shy	Helps me drink more when I'm up late at a club

Your Choices

Remember, everyone is unique. You might have a different experience from anyone else. Then again, all of these drugs release dopamine to a greater or lesser degree, which makes you feel good. You have made choices about which drugs you use, too. And we know that those choices were made, at least initially, because you *like* how the drug makes you feel or you experience other positive things. You can use the simple chart on page 40 to

> Remember, everyone is unique.

reflect on the benefits of your own choices of drugs (or see the end of the Contents for information about downloading and printing your own).

What's Next?

Cheryl, Tyler, and Ruben have reasons for using the drugs they do in the ways they do. So do you. You can see that they are developing problems. You might be too, with at least one of your drugs. It is why you are reading this book. In the next chapter we will go more deeply into the *potential* harms that come from various drugs and the harms that you might be experiencing. This is where harm reduction gets complicated. You will need to be precise about the details of your use if you are to reduce harm and avoid hysteria. We will do our best to help you avoid hysteria so that you can make calm and rational decisions about what to change, and when.

Drug use is ubiquitous in almost all human societies as far back as we can know.

Not all drug use is misuse.

Drugs work!

My Choices

Drug	Why I Started Using	Why I Use Now

3 When Is Drug Use Harmful?

The poison is in the dose.
—Attributed to PARACELSUS,
16th-century Swiss-German physician

There is a fine line between a medicine and a poison. In the right doses, plant-based drugs (alcohol, opioids, morning glories, mushrooms, or cannabis—marijuana to us older folks) and laboratory-produced drugs (methamphetamine, ecstasy, ketamine, or LSD) can deliver life-changing medicine or mood-enhancing experience. Take too much and you can die, develop a chronic illness, kill someone else, or wreck your or your family's life. How much is too much? *It depends*. This chapter will introduce you to how to analyze how much is too much for *you*.

Harm comes not only from a substance itself but also from society's response to certain drugs. As often stated by Ethan Nadelmann of the Drug Policy Alliance, "More harm has been done by the *War* on Drugs than was ever done by the *use* of drugs" [emphasis ours]. The fact that in America we have deemed certain drugs illegal (most of which are less harmful than the legal ones, alcohol and tobacco) means that millions of Americans have lost their families, their livelihoods, and in many cases their freedom.

Harm also comes from the secrecy that surrounds the use of illegal drugs—the fact that they are produced in labs that have no quality control and could contain any toxic substance, the fact that they are often consumed quickly in unclean conditions, and the fact that the dosage of the active ingredient is always uncertain means that millions of drug users risk serious consequences with each episode of use. As we write, drug users are being harmed by drugs that are not what they say they are. Produced in factories all over the world, an ecstasy pill might be anything but. Recently heroin has contained large amounts of fentanyl, a much stronger opioid, which has caused thousands of overdoses. And synthetic marijuana, such as K2 or Spice, or "designer" drugs such as bath salts can cause severe psychotic reactions.

Finally, harm comes from the fact that we usually pay attention only to "addiction" or prohibition. In so doing, we miss the opportunity to give people, including and especially teenagers, real and scientific information about drugs—the benefits *and* the risks. In their ignorance of this information, people are much more likely to get into trouble with the most innocent of experiments.

Drugs are complicated. Not only do they have benefits, but they also cause harm. Harm is what we usually focus on—*over*drinking and virtually any use of other drugs are deemed alcoholism or addiction. We gave you a chapter on benefits before this one so that you could get firmly grounded in your reasons for using *that make sense*. Harm almost always comes after, sometimes long after, one has enjoyed the benefits of using.

> Harm almost always comes after one experiences the benefits of using drugs.

Even after harmful effects emerge, a drug can continue to be useful. Harm reduction pays attention to the nuances of each person's unique relationship with drugs and to each person's situation. The associate attorney working 80 hours a week downs a few whiskeys on weeknights to relieve tension because there is no time for the gym. It is only after three cups of coffee the next morning that he is on his game again. On weekends, however, he runs, plays tennis, and has dinner with the woman he is dating. Over dinner they share a bottle of great wine. Whiskey never crosses his mind. *Harm is also highly personal.* Another attorney, also working long hours, is shy and not particularly athletic. He continues to drink throughout the weekend and ends up staying at home watching TV. He may or may not be drinking *more* than the first person, but he is more likely to suffer as a result of his drinking because alcohol holds a more central place in his life.

Harm is relative. **It depends.** This chapter will help you begin to sort out whether or not your use is harmful for *you*. Here you might run into information that you have been avoiding. It's not easy to look closely at the details of your drug use for fear of discovering something you didn't want to know. So take it slow. Put the book down for now if you're not ready to focus on the problems you're experiencing. Come back later.

Do You Have to Be an *Addict* to Be Harmed?

No! And this tired old word is full of judgment and stigma. It draws a sharp line between use and misuse and creates a dichotomy that draws our attention to addiction or to illegal use, regardless of whether that use is harmful. It precludes the reality that the same drug in the same amount can become harmful for one person and not another, that neither of these people needs to be considered (or be) an addict, and that harm can coexist with benefits. Finally, it's hard to take an honest look at yourself when you start out feeling like a second-class citizen!

What *is* true is that harm can occur with *any* use of drugs or alcohol, not just "addictive" use. The (primarily) young men who have died during fraternity drinking bouts at colleges were probably not dependent on alcohol. Although they were drinking way too heavily on those occasions, they may not have been chronic or heavy drinkers in general. In fact, if they *had* been regular heavy drinkers, they might *not* have died: their ability to tolerate large amounts of alcohol, to "handle their liquor," would have been stronger. They died because they drank more than their central nervous system could tolerate.

The (primarily) young women raped at college drinking parties are probably not "alcoholic." They are participating in a drunken ritual called a college party. They

> Harm can occur with any use of drugs or alcohol, not just "addictive" use.

might also be mixing drugs, whether knowingly or not. Under the influence of alcohol, they become a commodity to be used and abused.

In the same way, your first experiment with heroin could be your last. You meant no harm; you just didn't have *tolerance*—your body's ability to handle (adapt to) the effects of drugs that increase the more you use. (When people say they can "hold their liquor," they are talking about tolerance.) Most people know by now that a single dose of heroin or speed, if injected with a shared needle, can result in HIV or hepatitis C. Experimenting just that one time can mean risking serious, possibly lifelong, harm. Typically, ecstasy is used on an occasional social basis, not in a frequent "addictive" pattern. But it may still cause depression during withdrawal. And if you mix it with too much alcohol and too little water when you're dancing, it can cause fatal kidney failure due to dramatically high body temperature.

So, no, you don't have to be an "addict" to be harmed. And you can prevent harm by knowing what you are using and how to use it. Harm is an individual thing. **It depends.**

The Continuum of Drug Use

Most people use alcohol and other drugs—occasionally or routinely—without suffering significant harms and without misusing. We've been told by the press, by some professionals, by our parents, and by lawmakers that drug use is dangerous and that experimentation is the first step down the road to ruin. But this dichotomous paradigm is misleading because it makes all use seem dangerous. This is not only inaccurate, but if the goal is to scare us away from using, it hasn't worked. And by denying accurate information about drugs to people who are going to use, regardless of what anyone says, we expose them to far greater risk than necessary.

In harm reduction, we think of your drug use on a *continuum* from occasional to moderate to heavy to chaotic (out of control) rather than an "I am or I'm not" dichotomy. We'll help you focus on what you use, how much, and whether you have risk factors to consider—an illness, emotional vulnerability, or other complicating factors—that would make your use of a drug heavy when for someone else it might be moderate. We identify the specific risks of each drug so that you can evaluate. Finally, we help you put it all together, to figure out the pattern of use for each of your drugs. Each pattern might have harms associated with it, but in general, the farther up the stairs you go in the picture on page 45, the more likely you are to encounter harm. The continuum that we use has been developed over the years by combining information from the Harm Reduction Coalition and from various writers in the harm reduction field.

> Denying accurate information about drugs to people who are going to use, regardless of what anyone says, exposes them to far greater risk than necessary.

Steps in the Continuum

No Use

You do not use psychoactive substances. Depending on your culture or your health, you may or may not count coffee, tea, or chocolate as psychoactive.

Experimental

You are curious about the effects of a drug or you are with people who invite you to get high with them. You use once or a few times. You don't maintain a supply.

Occasional

You may or may not have a particular pattern. You use occasionally at parties, events, or holidays—cocktails after work or beer watching a football

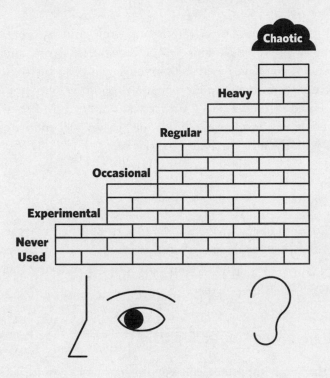

game, "poppers" (amyl nitrite) during sex, ecstasy at a dance club, or other people's cigarettes. You also *don't use* at events where others are because you don't feel like it. You use alone for a particular effect, such as smoking pot to make reading science fiction more interesting.

Regular

Using becomes more predictable. A pattern has been established. You go out drinking every weekend. You smoke weed whenever you're stressed from work, and that's about every other day. Or maybe it's once a month. Otherwise, you smoke when you're with friends at a party. You snort meth when you go to clubs, and that's almost every weekend except when you visit your parents. You take pills or shoot heroin every day. You may use recreationally, or your drug or drugs might be serving as an emotional "crutch" (*coping mechanism* is the term we prefer).

Heavy

Here is where *it depends*. "Heavy" depends on your health, on the norms of your group or culture, and on whether you have complicating emotional or medical issues that make your choice of drug riskier. Simply put, you use more than you "should." This evaluation is often a confusing and very subjective one. If you have hepatitis C, two beers is probably more than you "should" drink. If no one else in your social group smokes pot every day, you might be considered a heavy user if you do, but not if they do. Daily heroin use could be considered "regular" or "heavy" depending on whether it interferes with the other activities in your life.

Chaotic

Chaotic is the word that harm reduction uses to describe what most people mean when they say "addiction." You use heavily, your focus is dominated by your drugs, your life is unraveling, and you are suffering mental, emotional, or physical harm.

Safe, Moderate, and Controlled Use

These are the most important concepts in harm reduction. They are the goals that most people we know strive for. Any of the patterns of use above, with the likely exception of chaotic, can be controlled. All, including chaotic, can be safe. Occasional or regular use can be moderate. Standards of moderate alcohol use have been developed by an organization called Moderation Management (*www.moderation.org*), and responsible drinking standards have been published by the U.S. government (*www.rethinkingdrinking. niaaa.nih.gov*). Other resources are books like *Responsible Drinking* and the Responsible Drinking website (*www.responsibledrinking.org*); the Guided Self-Change program (*www.nova.edu/gsc/index.html*); CheckUp and Choices (*www.checkupandchoices.com*); and the HAMS network (Harm Reduction, Abstinence, and Moderation Support), which puts all options for drinking in one very flexible and supportive program (*www.hamsnetwork.org*).

Drug users can and do infer their own standards of moderate use from these guidelines. While heavy use falls outside the bounds of moderate, it can still be intentional, controlled, and safe—getting drunk at a wedding or a wake, really really stoned at a concert, intensely high on LSD, or totally tweaked out at a party. The medical, psychological, and relationship risks associated with heavy use can be evaluated using a cost/benefit analysis, and you have the right to enjoy yourself as you wish. Regardless of your pattern, you can still protect your safety and that of others. Throughout the rest of this book, we will refer often to safety, moderation, and control.

Substance Use Disorders and Substance Misuse

The American Psychiatric Association renamed the disorders formerly called *substance abuse* and *substance dependence* as *substance use disorders* and created subcategories of *mild, moderate,* and *severe*. This is a better categorization than abuse and dependence because it allows for a gradual evolution along the continuum of severity. There are a total of 11 symptoms in four categories (impaired control, social impairment, risky use, and pharmacological criteria), and the more symptoms you have, the more severe your substance use. Examples of symptoms include:

- You continue to use despite negative consequences (such as a DUI, missing work, getting into fights, depleting your bank account).

- You might be physically dependent. In other words, you have developed tolerance to the drug (your body has adapted to the drug), and you go into withdrawal if you stop.

- You crave your drugs and go out of your way to get them.

- Your life becomes organized around using.

- You try to cut back or quit and can't.

We and others in the harm reduction world use the term *substance misuse* to describe use that has become problematic. We find that it is a more neutral term than the more commonly used term *abuse* and adequately captures problems with substances. It also avoids the medical term *disorder*. The advantage of having the descriptive and plain-spoken terms *use* and *misuse* in our continuum is that we can be more precise. For example, heavy and chaotic use would certainly qualify as patterns of misuse. Regular use of one drug or another might qualify as misuse, too, if it incurs negative consequences. So could occasional use, if it is used in such a way as to cause an accident or overdose.

You might have had some thoughts about where your drug use falls along the continuum as you read the preceding descriptions. But what if you use more than one drug, as many of us do? We've learned that, contrary to the theory of "cross-addiction," people are often at different points on the continuum with each drug they use (see the box on the next page).

Where Do You Fall on the Continuum?

Let's say, for example, you use four different drugs: alcohol, cocaine, pot, and caffeine.

The Myth of Cross-Addiction

The concept of cross-addiction suggests that if you are in trouble with one drug, you'll have trouble with any. We've found, however, that each drug people use might be in a different category on the continuum. Most treatment programs insist that people abstain from all substances that are potentially "addictive," not just their drug of choice. This is because of fear of cross-addiction. Yet in an analysis of a large-scale study of substance misuse, a modest minority (13%) of people who resolved one substance use disorder developed another. (People who were more vulnerable to developing another substance use disorder were male, younger, never married, younger when they developed a problem, and suffering from a co-occurring psychiatric condition.) There has been some speculation that the specter of cross-addiction could be a self-fulfilling prophecy, at least for some individuals. This would fall in line with research on the abstinence violation effect—the belief that "one drink leads to 1,000" increases the likelihood that it will be so.

- Alcohol: You drink socially and on the light side, never more than two drinks a few times a week. This is occasional use. Or, you don't drink alcohol every day, but when you do you drink *a lot,* black out, drive your car, and generally cause mayhem. That's chaotic use.

- You use cocaine occasionally (once a month), but when you do, you party for the whole weekend, sometimes missing work on Monday. This falls into the heavy category.

- Your pot use is more confusing. You smoke just a little every day, and you need it to relax. When you smoke, though, whatever other good ideas you had for the evening—doing your taxes, writing the paper that's due next week, cleaning the garage—vanish. You've been trying to cut down, but it's not really working. This could be heavy use or a substance use disorder.

- You may be physically dependent on caffeine, needing two or three big cups to get you going in the morning. That's "regular" on the continuum (with physical dependence thrown in). (Notice we're not using the term *addicted*?)

To figure out where your drug use falls along the continuum, fill out the worksheets on pages 51–52, using one for each drug you use. We've supplied two copies here (see the end of the Contents for information on printing out additional copies). Notice, for example, the "complicating factors" are what we mentioned in the "heavy" section earlier in this chapter—things like drinking when you have hepatitis C or using way more than any of your friends do. Complications are anything else in your life that would affect, or be affected by, your drug use. We have filled out worksheets for Cheryl, Tyler, and Ruben as examples.

Continuum of Drug and Alcohol Use Worksheet: Examples

Cheryl

Drug	Amount	Frequency	Complicating Factors	Level of Use
Alcohol	4–5 glasses of wine	5 nights/ week	Trauma	Heavy
Opioid pills	2–4 pills	Daily		Regular/ heavy (physical dependence)

Tyler

Drug	Amount	Frequency	Complicating Factors	Level of Use
Speed	100 mg, and up to ½ gram on weekends	Daily	Loneliness	Regular/ chaotic on weekends
Alcohol	4 drinks on weekdays, up to 12 on weekends	Daily	Long-standing habit Loneliness	Regular/ chaotic on weekends

Ruben

Drug	Amount	Frequency	Complicating Factors	Level of Use
Ecstasy	2 pills	Once a week	Loneliness	Regular
Alcohol	5–10 drinks	3–4 nights a week	HIV	Heavy

Drug	Amount	Frequency	Complicating Factors	Level of Use
Marijuana	4–5 "bowls"	Daily	Long-standing habit	Heavy
Cocaine	Up to 1 gram	3–4 nights a week	Depression and anxiety	Heavy/chaotic

Now take the information for each drug you entered into the worksheets and plot your drug use on the worksheet on page 53 (or see the end of the Contents for information on printing out additional copies). Enter the name/s of your drug/s on the appropriate step and, in the blanks "under" the steps, write in the amount, frequency, and complicating factors. In this way, you can see at a glance where your drugs belong on the continuum. As your use changes, you can revise this again and again. (It will be easiest to do this if you use the form available online. Because you may want to add more information as suggested later in the chapter, if you decide to print the form and fill it out by hand, be sure to print it out full size, so it fills a whole page of paper.)

Harm

There's no doubt that drug use carries some risk. And because drug use is risky, harm can come to anyone who uses drugs or alcohol. Lest you sink into self-recrimination, let us remind you that many other things carry risk, too—skiing, mountain climbing, working 70 hours a week, eating large amounts of red meat, driving a car, or getting pregnant. So is your drug use harmful? It depends. As you reflected on in Chapter 2, it's likely that your use of drugs was at first a solution for something, but perhaps now it has become the problem.

How do we define harm? Let's start by favoring complexity over simplicity. If we simplify the definition of *harm* for a particular set of circumstances, we're likely to overlook important complicating factors—"wild cards"

> Many other things carry risk. So is your drug use harmful? It depends.

that have the power to turn risk into harm. Let's say you're not dependent on alcohol, but you have diabetes. You drink beer twice a week. Is that safe? Not necessarily—it could be lethal. Let's say you have high blood pressure and you use cocaine just once. Is it safe? Maybe, but stroke is a risk for

Continuum of Drug and Alcohol Use Worksheet

Drug	Amount	Frequency	Complicating Factors	Level of Use

Continuum of Drug and Alcohol Use Worksheet

Drug	Amount	Frequency	Complicating Factors	Level of Use

My Continuum of Drug and Alcohol Use

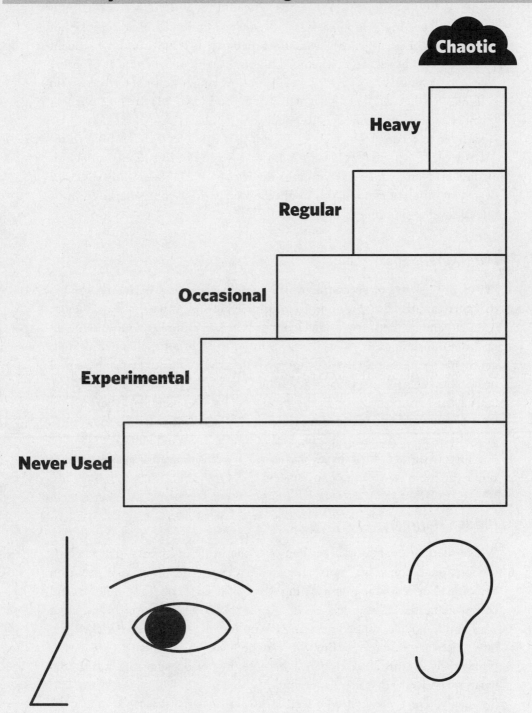

cocaine use *and* high blood pressure. Or you're a student, and you smoke pot once a week or so. Marijuana can affect memory. Is it harmful for a student who is not "addicted" to marijuana to use it? Maybe, maybe not. It probably

> It's the "wild cards" that can create the conditions for harm to occur.

depends on how much he or she smokes and when. Is it a good idea? Maybe not, but that also depends.

It's not that any one of these things is *the truth*. It's that if you try to simplify a drug or alcohol problem, you're likely to miss the *interaction* and the *relative importance* of several different factors. You might then apply the wrong solution or miss one of several solutions.

Harm versus Risk

Harm and risk are often confused. Risk involves *potential* harm and implies that there are things we can do to minimize getting in harm's way. We use seat belts and helmets, triple-check our gear before climbing a mountain, get up from our desk chair to stretch for 5 minutes each hour, change our diet, get prenatal care. Sure, taking drugs can pose a risk of health problems, social or vocational problems, or overdose. But taking risks is not necessarily the problem. *Ignoring* the risks and failing to take precautions is what causes harm. Let us not forget, though, that harm can also simply be the tragic result of an accident.

> It's not taking risks that's the problem. It's ignoring the risks and not taking precautions that causes harm.

Hidden Harm

While there are harms that hit you over the head and harms that become obvious once you learn more about your drugs—the impact of wine on hepatitis C or marijuana on learning—not all harm is obvious. The painful hangover headache, the despair after your spouse leaves you, the fact that your children have stopped speaking to you or your parents have kicked you out—these are easy to see. But you may be incurring harms that are not so visible. We call this "hidden harm" because the person who suffers from the harm is not aware that it is occurring.

Say you're a teenager who feels awkward in social situations (and what teen doesn't?). You may experiment with alcohol and discover that drinking increases your confidence, makes you witty and fun to be around. You use Molly so you can dance with abandon, even though at other times you think you're a horrible dancer. What's the harm in it? You don't drive after you've been drinking, and ill effects you feel the next day after a night of E are tolerable. The hidden harm might be that you don't ever get to practice being yourself around other people, to tolerate *not* being totally cool, to learn that anxiety won't kill you, and to enjoy dancing regardless of how uncoordinated you are. This missed experience can keep you tied to drinking and drugs long after you want to be.

Maybe you're a musician or an artist who finds that marijuana relaxes you so that ideas flow more smoothly, the music dances off your fingertips. And so you use it, and you produce art. The hidden harm may show up a few years down the road, when you discover that your creations are good but you haven't really produced anything marketable. Or you've produced a finished piece but just can't quite get yourself an agent, so no one gets to see it. You've tolerated the obvious harms of smoking marijuana—your girlfriend's nagging, the way your physique has lost its edge, occasional lapses of memory—but this hidden harm to your career takes you by surprise.

You might have been molested as a child. You began to dissociate, a more extreme version of "checking out"—to mentally leave your body to get away from the horrible thing that's happening to you. The problem is, you don't always have control over when it happens, so you miss important things, like what your teacher is saying or vital portions of a meeting. You discover that heroin or alcohol allows you to check out too. It quiets the demons that haunt you. The risks of heroin and alcohol are no mystery. (Their advantages to victims of abuse, however, are not given nearly enough credit.) What is less obvious is the lack of emotional development you experienced during the years that you were checking out. We've heard thousands of people say, once they started examining their relationship with drugs, "I feel like I'm still 15 years old, like I missed growing up with regular emotions."

In the following section, in the spirit of Just Say Know, we offer you a brief list of risks and harms of each major class of drugs.

Harms Minus the Hysteria

There is a comprehensive section on drugs at the end of this book. But we want to offer you a quick look at the potential harms of different drugs, harms that are *real,* not based on fear: harms minus the hysteria. We have organized this brief information by physical, behavioral, and psychological harm.

A general note: Mixing drugs raises your potential for danger. If they are both sedating, then you risk overdose. If you use multiple stimulants, you increase the risk of heart attack and stroke. If you mix sedating and stimulant drugs, they mask each other's effects and you risk taking too much of either.

Alcohol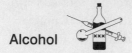

PHYSICAL

- Alcohol affects more organ systems than any other drug—liver, heart, brain, pancreas, kidneys, and digestive system (by interfering with the absorption of nutrients).

- In large amounts at one time, it can cause alcohol poisoning, which can be fatal.

- Stopping drinking suddenly can cause dangerous withdrawal, including seizures and DTs (delirium tremens).

- Disruption of the natural sleep cycle (even though people often use alcohol to *get* to sleep).

BEHAVIORAL

- Accidents and violence are the most common harms caused by alcohol use, and alcohol is implicated in 50% of arrests in the United States.

- The disinhibiting effects of alcohol can lead to errors in judgment and inappropriate behaviors like saying things you regret, TWD (texting while drunk), or having unwanted or unsafe sex, especially during a blackout.

PSYCHOLOGICAL/COGNITIVE

- Anxiety and/or depression (though the subjective experience is often relief from emotional suffering).

- At late stages, alcohol dementia.

Cannabis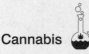

PHYSICAL

- Loss of coordination.
- May cause lung damage with heavy smoking.

BEHAVIORAL

- You are *not* a better driver under the influence of cannabis, even if you think you are.

> If you think you drive better when stoned . . . you must be high!

PSYCHOLOGICAL/COGNITIVE

- Some people become paranoid after using.

- Correlation between chance of developing schizophrenia and heavy teenage use; this research is controversial because it is difficult to know if teenagers who use more are predisposed and are self-medicating.

- Concentration and memory problems.

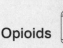

Opioids

PHYSICAL

- Risk of overdose.

- Physical tolerance and dependence, which causes very difficult withdrawal.

- Risk of contracting HIV, hepatitis, and infections with intravenous heroin use.

BEHAVIORAL

- Accidents and injuries.

- Victimization when "nodding out."

PSYCHOLOGICAL

- Anxiety, depression, and low self-esteem as a result of a lifestyle of danger and secrecy, and the stigma of being a "junkie."

Stimulants

PHYSICAL

- Increased blood pressure, stroke, and heart attack.

- Jitteriness.
- Reduces flow of saliva, which can cause gum and tooth decay.

BEHAVIORAL

- Engaging in high-risk behaviors, including sex without protection.
- Repetitive compulsive behaviors (picking, cleaning, counting).

PSYCHOLOGICAL

- Anxiety.
- Depression in withdrawal.
- Paranoia and psychosis with long-term use.

Sedatives/Hypnotics

PHYSICAL

- Physical tolerance and dependence. Stopping suddenly can cause dangerous withdrawal, including seizures.
- Risk of overdose when mixed with alcohol.

BEHAVIORAL

- Impaired driving.
- Injuries from falling or bumping into things.

PSYCHOLOGICAL/COGNITIVE

- Can impair short-term memory and new learning.

Nicotine

PHYSICAL

- Most of the following negative physical effects come from the tobacco "delivery system" (smoking or chewing), not from nicotine itself:
  - Lung problems, including emphysema and cancer.
  - Cancers of the mouth and throat.

- Increased blood pressure.
- Premature aging of the skin.

BEHAVIORAL

- Considered an antisocial behavior these days; risk of ostracism.

PSYCHOLOGICAL

- Reduced self-esteem from the stigma of being a smoker.

Entheogens

The possible harms associated with this class of drugs are different for each group.

Hallucinogenic or Psychedelic Drugs

LSD, psilocybin mushrooms, peyote, and ayahuasca, for example.

PHYSICAL

- Nothing notable.

BEHAVIORAL

- Nothing notable.

PSYCHOLOGICAL

- Anxiety or panic, aka bad trips.
- Flashbacks.

Ecstasy

PHYSICAL

- Overheating and dehydration if used during strenuous activity with too little water.

BEHAVIORAL

- Dancing too hard and drinking too little water at parties.

PSYCHOLOGICAL

- Depletion of serotonin: post-high depression and lethargy.

Dissociative Anesthetics—Ketamine, PCP, Dextromethorphan

PHYSICAL

- Traumatic injuries.

BEHAVIORAL

- Being victimized due to not paying attention to surroundings.
- Aggression (PCP).

PSYCHOLOGICAL

- Panic, feeling out of one's body.
- Difficulty recovering a sense of reality.

Deliriants/Inhalants

These drugs include household solvents, gasoline, glue, butyl nitrate, and nitrous oxide.

PHYSICAL

- Brain damage due to lack of oxygen.
- Death by asphyxiation (sudden inhalant death).
- Loss of muscle control leading to falls and accidents.
- Lung damage from contamination.
- Permanent damage to motor system of brain.

BEHAVIORAL

- Excessive risk taking.
- Aggression.

PSYCHOLOGICAL

- Paranoia.
- Severe cognitive impairments: memory, concentration.
- Unpredictable mood swings.

Designer/Synthetic Drugs

New drugs are continually under development in order to avoid drug laws. The list is endless. Current examples are bath salts, Spice, and 2CB. Some are hallucinogens, some are attempts at synthetic marijuana, and some are primarily stimulants. In the case of synthetic cannabinoids, it is not clear what they are mixed with, and people are at risk of seizures and death due to respiratory depression.

"Pills" could be anything these days. Because so many are manufactured for the drug market in unregulated factories in other countries or in home labs, they are unlikely to be true Vicodin, Valium, or oxycodone, which is often what people are seeking. Recent lab tests have found up to 12 substances in one pill. If you don't know what the drugs are, you have no way of anticipating what the effects are going to be.

If you have found information about your drugs that is of use to you, expand the continuum worksheets you filled out earlier, this time adding the harms and risks that you incur. These examples and the blank worksheet on page 62 illustrate how your worksheets will look.

| Harms/Risks of Drug and Alcohol Use Worksheet: Examples |

Cheryl

Drug	Amount	Frequency	Complicating Factors	Level of Use	Harms/Risks
Alcohol	4–5 glasses of wine	Almost daily	History of sexual abuse	Heavy	Causes fights with boyfriends Hard to get up for work on Monday

Harms/Risks of Drug and Alcohol Use Worksheet

Drug	Amount	Frequency	Complicating Factors	Level of Use (guess)	Harms/Risks

Tyler

Drug	Amount	Frequency	Complicating Factors	Level of Use	Harms/Risks
Speed	Smokes all day and night— not sure how much	Every weekend	Stressful job	Heavy	Drink more when I use Sometimes miss work on Monday Depressed the next day

Ruben

Drug	Amount	Frequency	Complicating Factors	Level of Use	Harms/Risks
Alcohol	5–10 drinks	3–4 nights a week	HIV	Heavy	Possible liver problems when mixed with HIV meds
Marijuana	4–5 "bowls"	Daily	Long-standing habit	Heavy	Trouble concentrating at work

Again, if you would like, add this additional information about your relationship with drugs to the My Continuum of Drug and Alcohol Use worksheet on page 53 (or see the end of the Contents for information on printing out additional copies—if you print it to fill it out by hand, make sure you print it as a full page to have enough space).

Cost/Benefit Analysis: Putting It All Together

Harm can be thought of as the *cost* that you pay. But as you clarified in the last chapter, you also *benefit* from each of your drugs. Now we invite you to put it all together and see your patterns, the benefits, and the costs of each drug. Our goal is to help you understand the conflicts that you are struggling with, the interplay of the benefits that you get and the harms that you are suffering.

Pull out the benefits that you wrote down in Chapter 2 and the harms that you identified in this chapter and add them to the worksheet on page 65 (see the end of the Contents for information on printing out additional

copies). First you may want to look at the examples from Cheryl, Tyler, and
Ruben that appear below.

Benefits and Harms of Drug and Alcohol Use Worksheet: Examples			

Cheryl

Drug	Level of Use	Benefits	Risks/Harms
Alcohol	Regular	Great sex Can't think of any better way to relax after my day at work	Causes fights with boyfriends Hard to get up for work on Monday

Tyler

Drug	Level of Use	Benefits	Risks/Harms
Speed	Heavy	Makes social situations less awkward and more exciting	Drink more Sometimes miss work Depressed the next day

Ruben

Drug	Level of Use	Benefits	Risks/Harms
Alcohol	Heavy	Helps me relax socially	Possible liver problems when mixed with HIV meds
Marijuana	Heavy	Helps me block out painful memories	Trouble concentrating at work

If you'd like, put it all together in the My Continuum of Drug and
Alcohol Use worksheet on page 53 (or see the end of the Contents for information on printing out additional copies); again, if you print it out to fill in
by hand, be sure to print as a full page).

We hope you now have a good idea of how your drug use impacts your
life, for better and for worse.

Benefits and Harms of Drug and Alcohol Use Worksheet

Drug	Level of Use	Benefits	Risks/Harms

What's Next?

Now that you have a pretty good idea of the level of your use, the benefits, and the risks or potential harms of each drug, we invite you in the next two chapters to deepen your understanding of the interaction between yourself, your drugs, and the context in which you use. The next chapter will introduce a model called "Drug, Set, Setting," which allows you to take into account *all* of the complexities of you, your use, and the world you live in. Adding your unique life circumstances will help you create a picture of the real, complicated you. That way, any changes you might decide to make will be defined and directed by you. As always, if you want to shut it down, or turn to someone else for help, either close the book or turn to Chapter 11.

You might suffer harm from one drug but not another.

Even after harmful effects have emerged, a drug can continue to be helpful.

It's not taking risks that's the problem—it's not taking precautions to prevent harm.

4 Why Do Some People Get into Trouble While Others Don't?

It's not the drugs, it's the need to escape reality.
—Anonymous

Why do some people drink or use drugs without problems while others run into trouble at every turn? First we need to define trouble. Essentially, trouble comes when we use "too much, too often." Or when we use drugs that fit poorly with our mental, emotional, or physical condition or with our surroundings. Trouble comes when your drugs interfere with what else you want to or should be doing.

In this chapter, we will present various theories about how some people get into trouble with drugs, while others don't. There is no single "truth" about problems with drugs. There are, however, three major theories—the disease model, learning theory, and the self-medication hypothesis—that have attracted the most attention. We also offer other theories that are less well known but are very important. We then explain the model that harm reduction is based on, the model that integrates all aspects of your relationship with drugs.

We offer you a variety of theories so that you can find the best way of understanding *your* relationship with drugs. You might also have your own theory. Pick and choose what makes sense and what will, ultimately, help you find your way out of trouble.

Major Theories

The Disease Model of Addiction

Elsewhere in the world called the American disease model, the basic belief is that people who misuse alcohol or other drugs have a physical disease. Before the 19th century, Benjamin Rush, a physician considered the father of American psychiatry, set about trying to understand "chronic drunkenness," which had up until then been considered a sin. Rush said that drunkenness acts "as if" it is a disease. He developed a "moral and physical thermometer" of alcoholism, in which he distinguished between "temperance" (what we now call moderation) and "intemperance," which led to vices such as lying, anarchy, and murder; diseases—puking and tremors, swelling of the legs, madness, and death; and such punishments as black eyes, the poorhouse, whipping post, and gallows. He set in motion more than a century of seeking a cure for dipsomania (alcoholism), including institutionalization, cold showers, toxic cocktails, and frontal lobotomies. Temperance movements of the 19th and early 20th centuries redefined temperance to mean abstinence from alcohol. Led by women (who suffered greatly from domestic violence and the loss of family income) and religious leaders in England and the United States, the temperance movement was entwined with women's suffrage, religious movements, and anti-immigrant sentiment.

In the United States, prohibition was instituted with the passage of the Eighteenth Amendment, which banned the manufacture, transportation, and sale of alcoholic beverages (but not its consumption, strangely) except for religious and medicinal use. Prohibition was a disaster. It inadvertently gave organized crime, which operated the majority of illegal import and sales of alcohol, its major foothold in the American economy. While Americans had previously consumed beer and wine, prohibition led to rapid drinking of hard liquor in underground bars (speakeasies), a pattern that was driven by fear of police raids. After 13 years, prohibition was repealed in 1933. Americans were again free to pursue explanations and cures for "alcoholism." The cure that took center stage was religious conversion, popularized by Bill Wilson, who founded Alcoholics Anonymous in 1935 after his own conversion experience. Thus alcoholism was reframed as a spiritual malady that required a religious conversion.

In the 1940s, alcohol researcher E. M. Jellinek was hired by an AA member to study alcoholism. His "disease concept of alcoholism" transformed the metaphor of the 18th century into truth of the 20th. Jellinek's subjects were a small group of AA members who voluntarily returned a questionnaire they saw in an AA magazine. This type of research, without a representative sample of all problem drinkers, is considered invalid. Nevertheless, his description lives on today, usually in this form: "addiction is a progressive incurable disease that ends in jails, institutions, and death." Unless, of course, the disease process is arrested by lifelong abstinence from psychoactive substances.

Since the 1990s, the field of neurobiology has laid claim to emotional and mental health conditions, including drug misuse, and they are now known as brain diseases. Conditions such as depression and schizophrenia became diseases that required medical, not psychological, interventions. So did problems with psychoactive drugs. The National Institute on Drug Abuse (NIDA) defines "addiction" as "a chronic, relapsing brain disease that is characterized by compulsive drug seeking and use, despite harmful consequences. It is considered a brain disease because drugs change the brain; they change its structure and how it works. These brain changes can be long lasting and can lead to many harmful, often self-destructive, behaviors." The emphasis is on the brain reward system—the idea that using psychoactive drugs activates dopamine, the primary brain chemical responsible for feelings of pleasure, thereby giving us the message "That feels good; do it again." According to the theory, thus begins the process of drugs "hijacking" the brain—consistent use causes changes in the brain reward circuitry activated by dopamine and in other brain areas related to memory and learning. These changes drive repeated use and the user becomes addicted.

Another aspect of the disease model concerns the role of genetic predisposition to drug misuse. What the data seem to show is that genetics play a variety of roles in a person's susceptibility to substance misuse. McLellan and colleagues found that genetic heritability, personal choice, and environmental factors are similarly involved in the cause and course of many chronic diseases, including substance use disorders. In other words, addiction is a chronic illness no different from diabetes, hypertension, or asthma. While we do not find the disease concept to be the best way of understanding substance misuse, we have great respect for the authors and we appreciate their demonstrating the shared influence of genetics, personal choice, *and* environment on the development of "addiction." Our experience says that the relative importance of these three factors is unique to each individual.

> Genetics, personal choice, and environment are all factors in substance misuse—their relative importance is unique to each individual.

We think the brain disease theory is oversimplified, confuses correlation with causality, and can't fully explain a complex problem; its flaws are discussed in the box on page 70. Many people (and institutions), however, find comfort in the disease model because it simplifies the problem, defining it as something that lies outside of our personal control and responsibility, something that is unaffected by the world in which we live. Diseases *happen* to people. Some fall ill and others don't.

Gaps Left by the Disease Model
of Substance Misuse

A Model of Inevitability

In their challenge to the monopoly of neuroscience in explaining addiction, among other mental health conditions, psychiatrist Sally Satel and psychologist Scott Lilienfeld explain brain disease theory as follows: Drugs stimulate the release of dopamine in the brain's reward circuits that also respond to food, sex, and other activities necessary for survival. Because dopamine floods us with feelings of pleasure, we are induced to repeat these behaviors and thereby survive and procreate. Drugs begin to inhabit the same important place as sex and food and overcome the parts of the brain that inhibit behavior. The problem, from the authors' point of view, is that most "addicts" do not use all the time. They spend much time doing other things. And they also decide to quit. In fact most quit in a natural process that others call "maturing out." By this reasoning, compulsive drug use is not a one-way street.

A Model of Pathology

Marc Lewis argues that what we call addiction is the brain acting in exactly the way it is supposed to: that is, to lead us to pleasurable and sustaining activities. Unfortunately, if our life doesn't offer such rewards, drugs will. Our brain then becomes very active in creating the sensations that cause overuse. These brain changes come about because of neuroplasticity—the brain's ability to change through experiences. But it's exactly this neuroplasticity that can be harnessed to rewire an "addicted brain," not through medications, but by creating experiences, skills, and a life that can provide more of the pleasures and satisfactions that we require.

Correlation versus Causation

There is no debate that drugs act on the brain, causing release of brain chemicals that induce pleasure, relaxation, stimulation, sharpening of perception, warm feelings, hallucinations, and so forth. That is, after all, the point! We take drugs precisely *because* they cross the blood–brain barrier and induce these experiences and feelings. Brain disease theory rests on brain scans, more precisely on how brain scans are *interpreted*. Brain scans measure activation (neuronal firing) and energy in the form of glucose. The problem is, *every* mental, emotional, and physical experience causes activation and energy flow in the brain. Furthermore, the brain is changed by all repeated actions. From childhood trauma (interpersonal and environmental) to malnutrition to lack of stimulation, brain development is affected. This means we can't isolate the effects of substance use from those of other repeated actions unless the brains of substance users have been observed *before* use ever begins.

It's Illogical

Just because drugs *impact* the brain doesn't mean that drug misuse *is* a brain disease any more than heavy drinking *is* liver disease. It is one *cause* of liver disease, but it is not, in and of itself, liver disease. Stanton Peele has been pointing out this logical misstep for more than 30 years.

On Genetics

Gene Heyman, a behavioral economist who has been studying addiction as a "disorder of choice," comments that *all* behavior has a genetic basis—including voluntary acts, for example, such as the selection of political party and religion (among the many likenesses discovered in identical twins separated at birth). "The brain is the organ of voluntary action."

It's Not Just Biology

The brain disease model assumes that neural processes are the primary drivers of our behavior. It gives little credit to environmental and interpersonal stress, pleasure seeking, medicinal use, or the many other reasons that people seek drugs and continue to use them.

The brain disease model also ignores the results of the Rat Park study (see the box on page 72–73), which pointed out the enormous role of environmental stress in compulsive substance use. In his chapter on Rat Park in *Chasing the Scream,* Johann Hari speculates that if we located the problem of drugs in poverty, violence, and trauma we would have to seek solutions that the United States lacks the political will to address.

If addiction is a disease, why are most of our "solutions" either punitive (jails and prisons) or based on faith in God or a higher power?

Even though NIDA proclaims addiction to be a brain disease, our zero-tolerance laws, attitudes, and treatments retain vestiges of the old moral model. People with substance use disorders are routinely called "liars" who have to be confronted with their "denial" or thrown in jail.

Rat Park

In the late 1970s Professor Bruce Alexander and colleagues at Simon Fraser University in Vancouver, British Columbia, decided to test the research showing that rats, given a choice of plain water and water laced with morphine, would choose the morphine and become addicted, thus proving that addictive drugs caused addiction. Alexander proposed three premises to challenge the research to date:

> First, the ancestors of laboratory rats in nature are highly social, sexual, and industrious creatures. Putting such a creature in solitary confinement would be the equivalent of doing the same thing to a human being. Solitary confinement drives people crazy; if prisoners in solitary have the chance to take mind-numbing drugs, they do. Might isolated rats not need to numb their minds in solitary confinement for the same reason that people do? Second, taking drugs in a Skinner box where almost no effort is required and there is nothing else to do is nothing like human addiction which always involves making choices between many possible alternatives. Third, rats are rats. How can we possibly reach conclusions about complex, perhaps spiritual experiences like human addiction and recovery by studying rats? Aren't we more complex and soulful than rats, even if we have similar social needs? (*www.brucekalexander.com/articles-speeches/rat-park/148-addiction-the-view-from-rat-park*)

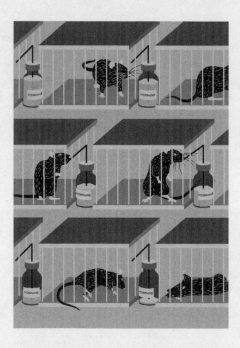

Alexander and his colleagues studied rats in a completely different kind of cage—they built a large wooden box full of tunnels, toys, and male and female rats. In other words they created an environment that approximated a rat's usual living situation. The rats played, had sex, and had babies. The researchers compared drug-taking behavior in Rat Park to that of rats who were in traditional laboratory cages as well as those who started life in traditional cages and then moved into Rat Park. The rats in Rat Park consumed far less morphine than the caged rats. This led Alexander to conclude that the environment is a more important determinant of addiction than the drugs themselves.

Two very informative and enjoyable summaries of Rat Park can be found in Stuart McMillen's cartoon (*www.stuartmcmillen.com/comics_en/rat-park*) and Johann Hari's TED talk (*www.ted.com/talks/johann_hari_everything_you_think_you_know_about_addiction_is_wrong*). As a result of his extensive interviews with Alexander and his reading of Alexander's work, Hari summed up his conclusions by saying, "The opposite of addiction is not sobriety; it's human connection."

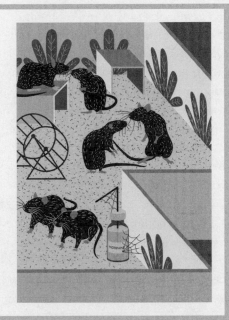

> Rats in Rat Park consumed far less morphine than caged rats. This means that environment is a more important determinant of "addiction" than the drugs themselves.

Learning Theory

Some substance use researchers and professionals believe substance misuse is a *learned behavior* that becomes habitual. Learning theories are psychological theories of how knowledge, behaviors, and skills are acquired and retained. Important concepts in learning theory are modeling (observing and imitating others), reinforcement (positive feedback or rewards), conditioned behavior (habits or patterns), and cognition (thoughts and beliefs).

For example, a person goes out for drinks one night after hearing his coworkers regaling each other with stories about last night's "blowout," and he decides to go along and see for himself (*modeling*). He then discovers that it relaxes him after a stressful day of work (*reinforcement*). After a few times, he realizes that he can count on this way of relaxing, so he develops a regular habit of stopping by the bar every day after work (*he has been conditioned*). Drinking provides pleasure and stress relief so consistently that he comes to *believe* this is the only way to de-stress in the evening and therefore keeps it up (*cognition*). It is in this combination of the pleasurable, reinforcing aspects of drug use and seeing peers doing the same thing that we learn new habits. There is nothing wrong with habits—brushing our teeth, stretching before running, and kissing the kids good-bye in the morning are habits. Problems will emerge from this man's after-work drinking habit if he stops doing other things (going to the gym, talking to other friends, having his weekly dinner with his parents) and relies only on drinking to reduce stress at the end of the day. His tolerance will go up, so he'll have to drink more to get the same effect, and he'll start experiencing hangovers that make it hard to work.

> There is nothing wrong with habits!

The most recent contribution to the learning literature comes from Maia Szalavitz, who has spent much of her career investigating and writing about neuroscience, addiction, and the abuses of the treatment system. In her new book *Unbroken Brain* she has turned her attention to creating a theory that addiction is a combination of timing and learning. It isn't driven by brain changes that *follow* the taking of drugs. Instead, it is a developmental process rooted in the history of an individual, his or her life situation, upbringing, culture, traumas, and joys. When drugs enter people's lives at particular moments in time, and they learn that drugs can help soothe them or even solve other problems in their lives, addiction occurs. To Szalavitz, brain changes that accompany chronic drug use are just a part of the process. Just as the brain reacts and adapts to all new experiences, it reacts and adapts to drugs. She points out also that what we see as behaviors leading to addiction are often quite normal and beneficial in other areas of life. For example, "When starving, when in love, and when parenting, being able to persist, despite negative consequences—the essence of addictive behavior—is not a bug, but a feature." We would say that persistence indicates *strength* of character. Why not pursue an activity that has proved to be a solution to a problem?

> Addiction is a combination of timing and learning, a developmental process rooted in a person's history—his or her life situation, upbringing, culture, traumas, and joys.

The Self-Medication Hypothesis

Harvard psychiatrist Edward Khantzian introduced the concept of self-medication in the 1980s. Khantzian observed that people use drugs in an attempt to take care of emotional problems. Common among his patients were difficulties with self-care, self-esteem, relationships, and handling intense feelings like anger, love, and fear. He also believed that people don't choose drugs randomly but instead choose those that are uniquely suited to medicate the painful feelings with which they struggle. Users of opioid drugs, for example, are trying to numb feelings of rage and aggression. Stimulants appeal because of their ability to relieve depression, treat the symptoms of ADHD, and counteract the dulling effects of medications for bipolar and psychotic disorders. Even though there are obvious pharmacological links between particular feelings and different drugs, we have found that you can't predict which drug a person will turn to based primarily on which emotions the person is struggling with. In fact, research indicates that cultural habits and norms and drug availability are more likely than feelings to determine the drugs you use.

During our 40 years of working with people who use drugs, we have observed that people are more likely to get into trouble with drugs if they use because they *need* to rather than because they *want* to. This is supported by the fact that many more people with mental health disorders misuse drugs than those without: 8.6% of the overall population over age 12 misuse alcohol and/or drugs, compared to 25% of those with major mental illnesses such as depression, anxiety, schizophrenia, and bipolar disorder. And almost 50% of people with substance use disorders have a coexisting mental health disorder. The rate of substance misuse among people with histories of trauma, which we will discuss later in the chapter, is far higher even than these figures. And why not? Most "street" drugs began life as medicines, and most still are! Drugs enliven, soothe, and offer escape. The fact that they may also cause harm down the road doesn't negate the benefits that they offer.

Silencing the Inner Critic

In the same way Khantzian observed that people medicate painful feelings with drugs, psychoanalyst Leon Wurmser noticed among his patients who used drugs in the later part of the 20th century that they did not *lack control* over their drug use so much as they needed drugs to *release* them from the control of their overly critical internal voices. Alcohol, for example, does a great job of shutting up one's internal critic (even though that critic might wake up with a vengeance along with the following morning's hangover). Another psychoanalyst, Otto Fenichel, suggested that "the superego is that part of the mental apparatus that is soluble in alcohol." Some people call this the itty bitty shitty committee.

In the following section, we discuss models that are more inclusive of a wide variety of individual experiences.

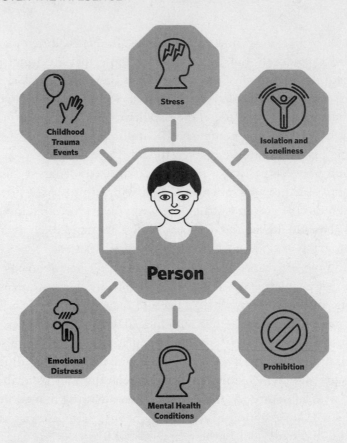

Other Important Theories of Substance Misuse

A Disorder of Choice

Psychologist Gene Heyman uses behavioral economics to seek a nondisease explanation for "persistent self-destructive drug use." Based on dozens of major surveys and studies of addiction, he has concluded that no other diseases are as "thoroughly caused" by voluntary behavior or can be eliminated entirely by voluntary behavior. Most striking is the fact that most people who have been addicted stop problematic substance use by the age of 30, and most do so without professional help. What kind of disease is that?

> Addiction is *not* a disease: no other diseases are as "thoroughly caused" by voluntary behavior or can be eliminated entirely by voluntary behavior.

People with *persistent* drug problems, Heyman found, tend to make choices based on "local" rather than "global optimum strategies." In other words, they pay more attention to their present situation and desired outcomes (relief from stress, recreation, social opportunities) and less attention to "global" choices that take into account the future, other people, their reputation, and so forth. So what looks like compulsive drug use might just be making choices based on present needs rather than future speculation.

The role of choice becomes less compelling when we look at the differences Heyman found between those who get over their addictions and those who don't. Those who quit are more likely to be married, have more years of education, be financially secure, have no additional psychiatric and medical problems, and be concerned about legal consequences and respect of family. Perhaps they had a lot to lose in the present if they continued problematic use, or they were guided more by global choices. People who *persist* in their addictive use beyond the age of 30, on the other hand, are more likely to have more co-occurring psychological problems, higher rates of medical disease, more crisis, more homelessness, fewer social supports, less money, less education, and fewer job opportunities. Perhaps they were making a logical choice when faced with short-term benefit versus the likelihood of long-term hopelessness. But, in fact, it might not feel like much of a choice at all. As Bruce Alexander, who discovered the importance of environment and stress in rats' "choice" to use or not use morphine, said, addiction may be a "choice in the absence of other options." To us, this seems closer to our clients' lived experience.

> There is a great deal of diversity among drug users and misusers. Some are intentional and happy about their choice. For others, perhaps we are talking about something more like forced choice, "choice in the absence of other options."

Vulnerability and Stress

Vulnerability refers to the soft spots, the gaps, in our psyches that leave us open to developing disorders, whether psychological or substance use disorders. Vulnerabilities can originate in genetics, our biology, psychology, or situation. Stress refers to events and circumstances that put sufficient pressure on us that it throws us off balance and disrupts our functioning. Each person has a unique set of vulnerabilities, which explains why each person is affected differently by the same or similar stressors (stressful events). The combination of our vulnerabilities and our life stress puts us at risk for developing a psychological disorder, including a problem with drugs.

Adverse Childhood Experiences

The largest study of the relationship between childhood trauma and the prevalence of illnesses in adulthood is the Adverse Childhood Experiences (ACE) study, summed up in the box below. Carried out by researchers at Kaiser Permanente and funded by the national Centers for Disease Control and Prevention, this study of 17,000 adults showed that ACEs are highly correlated with the leading 10 causes of death in the United States. Addiction was the second leading "illness" after chronic obstructive pulmonary disease (COPD). One of the study authors, Vincent Felitti, focused on what he calls "the origins of addiction." Data from his analysis of that part of the study are presented in the box.

The ACE study forces us to acknowledge the likelihood that family, community, and societal stresses play a larger role in the vulnerability

Results from the ACE Study

One point was assigned for one or more exposures to each of eight adverse childhood experiences: physical or sexual abuse, witnessing domestic violence, severe emotional abuse or neglect, having a parent with a severe drug problem or who has been incarcerated, or a parent with a severe mental disorder. In a follow-up study, emotional neglect was added.

- *Smoking*: People with an ACE score of 6 or higher had a 250% greater rate of smoking than people with no adverse childhood experiences.

- *Severe alcohol problem*: People with an ACE score of 6 or higher had a 500% greater rate of severe alcohol misuse than people with no adverse childhood experiences.

- *Injection drug use*: People with an ACE score of 6 or higher had a 4,600% greater rate of injection drug use than people with no adverse childhood experiences.

The study also analyzed the data for whether adverse childhood experiences could be considered to be *causes* of addiction; it determined that 67% of injection drug use overall (78% in the case of women) can be attributed to adverse childhood experiences.

As scores increase, there is a parallel increase in psychosocial problems, the adoption of high-risk behavior patterns (such as using drugs), chronic health problems, and premature death.

that leads to substance misuse than mere exposure to drugs and our brain chemistry. Felitti challenges the assumption that the brain changes inevitably brought on by the introduction of drugs into our systems are the *cause* of repeated and continued use. Just because drugs affect and bring about changes in the brain does not mean that there were not impairments beforehand. This challenge is supported by the brain research of trauma experts like Bessel van der Kolk showing that the brains of traumatized children are significantly different from those of nontraumatized children.

The ACE study creates a model whereby childhood experiences lead to impairments in social, cognitive, and emotional functioning. These impairments are partially or greatly relieved by using drugs, which in turn causes brain changes that solidify the tendency to continue using despite developing other problems. For example, Felitti cites numerous studies that demonstrate that nicotine moderates anger, anxiety, and hunger. And if, as we know, a child's endorphin system (the brain's opioid system) is impaired by traumatic experiences, why would one *not* seek opioid drugs in an attempt at repair? The ACE study supports both the learning and the self-medication theories of drug misuse. It supports both Bruce Alexander's and Marc Lewis's assertions that drugs take on important functions when a person has few opportunities in life for satisfaction, pleasure, or relief from emotional pain. And it allows for the impact of trauma on the brain and the further alterations in brain chemistry that help to drive drug use.

> The ACE study comes as close as anything we have ever read to explaining the real lives of the people we have worked with for dozens of years.

Problems in Attachment

One way of understanding drug use is that we become attached to our drugs in a way similar to our relationships with people. Whether they are permanent or fleeting, satisfying or unhappy, passionate or dull, they are relationships. *Harm reduction is based on the belief that there is a relationship between you, the user, and your drug of choice, in which the drug takes on many elements of a primary attachment figure.*

Research by John Bowlby beginning in the 1950s indicated that humans are hardwired to seek attachment to others, starting with primary caregivers at the beginning of life. The quality of those attachments leads to our style of relating to others as adults. With consistent care, attention, and nurturing, we grow up *secure* in our relationships. Disruptions in attachment (neglect, abuse, or abandonment) early in life create *insecure* relationship patterns (anxious, avoidant, or chaotic) that persist into adulthood. We are anxious and clingy, shy and avoidant, or unstable—we push and pull until we drive people away. Many others have followed in Bowlby's footsteps, and attachment theory has become central to the field of psychology. Following on Bowlby's work, Daniel Siegel, a leader in the growing field of interpersonal neurobiology, shows through brain imaging studies the specific brain structures that are negatively impacted by ruptures of attachment.

Both our relational experiences and their associated brain changes make us vulnerable to drug misuse, and our pattern of relating can even be reflected in the style of our drug use and misuse.

A therapist familiar with attachment theory, Karen Walant developed a cogent description of how attachment styles can lead to substance use problems and suggested treatment methods to address those attachment-related drug problems. She stressed that, in a society that values independence over dependency needs, children's needs for attachment are frustrated and they fail to develop a secure foundation, sometimes resulting in an attachment to things that are not human—such as drugs.

> In a society that values independence over dependency needs, children's needs for attachment are frustrated, sometimes resulting in an attachment to things that are not human—such as drugs.

Attachment theory is what inspired us to adopt the idea that people have a relationship with drugs. What we have learned over our 40 years of work in the field is that while drug use patterns, like relationships, exist on a continuum from healthy to seriously problematic, it is clear that serious problems are usually an expression of unmet needs from an earlier development period. We have learned from our clients who call alcohol the only friend they can count on, marijuana their antidepressant or antianxiety medicine, cocaine or speed their sex aid, opioids their warm blanket, and any drug in sufficient quantity their path to oblivion. A careful look at your history often reveals clear emotional or social problems for which you once actively sought solutions, then discovered drugs in your search. It is important for you, and those around you, to realize that drugs worked, at least a little, and at least for a while. This is one of those ideas that, once articulated, seems obvious and based in common sense. People are not stupid. We find what works and stick to it. The primary motivation is usually self-care, not self-destruction.

Cheryl, Tyler, and Ruben all have their own vulnerabilities that got them into trouble with drugs. Cheryl has a history of trauma that has left her unable to sustain an intimate relationship. Alcohol helps her relax enough to have sex. She is also berated by an inner critic so strict that she can't even tell her best friends she's also worried about her opioid pill use. Tyler is stuck in learned habits that have become entrenched. Despite the fact that he is getting into trouble at work, he is unable to change his use. He has an identity as a party animal, and his behavior fits that identity. He is also lonely and trying not to notice the emptiness in his life. Ruben is struggling with the trauma of childhood bullying and current loneliness.

Prohibition and Stigma

Prohibition refers to the actual laws that cause people to be incarcerated for drug use. Prisons are an obvious harm, both to the person in jail and to the family members who are forced to live without the jailed person. For example, when alcohol was made illegal for 13 years in the 1920s and early '30s many people went to prison, and those who continued to drink had to do so in secret clubs or make their own "bathtub gin," which was associated with severe medical problems. The enormous number of people incarcerated since the 1980s for illegal drug use has left thousands of children without the support of a parent or other relative. But prohibition is also felt internally. When we do things that we are told are wrong or illegal, we encounter stigma from the outside world but are also vulnerable to internalized stigma—shame and guilt.

Stigma kills. Being shunned, shamed, and ostracized is soul-destroying. It is not motivating; it is paralyzing. Being shunned and ostracized is about being excluded. It is humiliating. Shame is a feeling about oneself. It is different from guilt, which is a terrible feeling about something you *did,* and is often focused on the person or people you have wronged. Shame is feeling bad about *who or what you are*. It could be things about you that you probably can't change, like your race, a disability, or your family. Or it could be about something you did that you feel deeply ashamed of. Either way, the feeling is about you and how your actions reflect on the person you are. It is a feeling of being fundamentally flawed, and it is a very bad feeling. A feeling that begs to be eliminated by a strong dose of crack, speed, or heroin.

Someone in our community used to repeatedly scream when she was upset and high on speed, "SHAME DON'T CHANGE!" She was communicating something very important about the impact of shame on her drug use and the difficulty of changing anything about it. She and thousands like her are the reason that harm reduction is so radically accepting of people where they are. We welcome who you are, the choices you have made, and the drugs you use.

> Prohibition and stigma provide compelling reasons to get high—to eliminate the painful feelings of shame and guilt.

For an amazing explanation of Prohibition, check out Stuart McMillen's comic on the War on Drugs (*www.stuartmcmillen. com/comics_en/war-on-drugs*). In it, he covers the faulty rationale for the drug war and its impact on the health and wellness of drug users and society as a whole.

Why Some People Do Not Get into Trouble

Maturing Out, Self-Change, and Natural Recovery

To mature out of drug misuse means to get over it. It means moving on, walking away, evolving to other phases in one's life. As noted earlier, most people mature out of problematic drug use by the age of 30. Heyman says, "Addiction has the highest remission rate of any psychiatric disorder." Looking at different drugs, half of people who were dependent on cocaine remitted after 4 years, half of people who were dependent on marijuana had remitted after 6 years, and half of people with alcohol dependence after 16 years. These statistics are for people who did not go to treatment or self-help groups!

> Addiction has the highest remission rate of any psychiatric disorder.

Other researchers use the term *self-change* to mean change with no professional help. That does not, however, mean no help at all. The disappointment or disapproval of important people, suffering work performance, new responsibilities at work, marriage and children, and things that we cannot identify—that lie outside the realm of our consciousness—can contribute to transitioning out of heavy or problematic substance use. In other words, drug misuse simply becomes incompatible with one's current life roles and responsibilities. Some people also use *natural recovery*. But natural doesn't necessarily mean effortless. Changing patterns involves concentration, effort, enduring feelings of loss or deprivation, and getting up the nerve to fill one's time with new activities.

Resilience

Resilience means the ability to recover quickly from difficulties, to bounce back. People who are resilient are both strong and elastic (flexible). Think of the difference between glass and rubber if you throw a stone at it. The glass breaks. The stone bounces off the rubber. A major source of resilience is the presence of *protective factors*. Protective factors are characteristics inside and outside that make a person less likely to develop a substance use problem. The ACE study developed a list of questions to identify protective factors that help a child become resilient even in the face of adversity. Some of the experiences that build resilience include:

- Feeling like you were loved by at least one of your parents

- Having a parent or relative available to comfort you when you were upset

- Having reasonable rules at home that you had to keep

- Having a teacher or other adult point out your strengths

- Knowing that your parents cared about how you did in school

- If things were bad at home, having an adult you could confide in

Putting It All Together: A Biopsychosocial Perspective

Substance misuse is complicated, and harm reduction embraces this complexity. We have adopted a biopsychosocial model that takes everything into account—everything we've talked about in the previous section and more. This means that our *biology* (our body including our brain), our *psychology* (thoughts, beliefs, feelings, expectations, and motivations), and the *social context* in which we live and in which we use drugs interact in unique ways to create our experiences with drugs. We have adopted this model from Norman Zinberg, a psychiatrist and researcher at Harvard University, who developed a framework described in his book *Drug, Set, and Setting: The Basis for Controlled Intoxicant Use.*

While studying people who used heroin in the late 1970s and early 1980s, Zinberg discovered the phenomenon of recreational heroin use—people who had been using for years but hadn't become addicted. This went against the common belief that heroin, an "addictive" drug, automatically led to addiction. Through extensive interviews, he developed the understanding that addiction is not solely dependent on an "addictive" drug. Nor is it a matter of a person's being "diseased." What he found was that recreational heroin (and cocaine) users made the same sensible decisions that social drinkers do: there is a time and place for everything, and everything in moderation. Zinberg found that the key factor in controlled drug use was the existence of social controls. Social controls are a combination of social sanctions (the rules of conduct) and social rituals (patterns). Most people who drink, for example, do so within the social controls that govern alcohol use: "don't drink all day," "pace yourself," "know your limits," and "don't drink and drive" are among the many sanctions and rituals surrounding alcohol use.

> Controlled drug use is governed by social controls, of which there are plenty with regard to alcohol and tobacco, but many fewer in the use of other drugs because of their illegal status.

Zinberg proposed that the interactions between the *drug* (the pharmacological action of the substance itself—stimulant, sedative, psychedelic, and so forth), the *set* (the attitude or mind-set of the person at the time of use), and the *setting* (the physical and social setting in which a person uses) produce the effects of both recreational and problematic use.

Different mind-sets and settings influence the experience. For instance, a glass of wine with dinner is different from sharing a bottle of wine with a friend at happy hour, which is different again from drinking a bottle at home

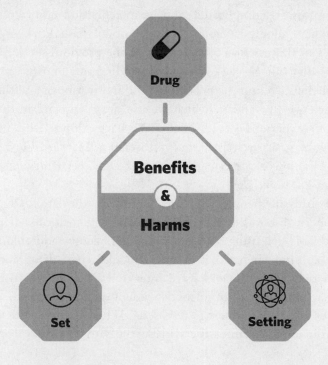

alone after a divorce and on an empty stomach. In the first case, wine is part of food, heightening the flavor and enjoyment of both. In the second, wine is both relaxing and intoxicating and enhances the pleasure of the other's company. In the third situation, enough wine will serve to dull pain and/or accentuate it, bringing on anger and tears. Not only do *problems* with drugs emerge, but often the *drug experience itself* is a product of this interaction. Your best experience on mushrooms was with your college roommates, and your worst trip ever was with a boyfriend you couldn't stand anymore. The speed that helped you stay up when you needed to study made you grind your teeth and pace the floor when you took it on Saturday morning so you could get to work at the restaurant. When you took it again Saturday night, you were so obnoxious that your friends asked you to leave. In other words, the same user can have different experiences, even with the same drug, on different occasions of use.

> The same user can have different experiences, even with the same drug, on different occasions of use.

In our work and in this book, we have taken some liberties with Zinberg's model. We have added details about the amount, frequency, route of administration, and legality of each drug used, as well as whether it is used in combination with other drugs or prescribed medications. We have included in our understanding of set a person's history (especially of trauma), gender identity, sexual orientation, ethnicity, other aspects of identity, personality, mental and emotional state, formal diagnosis of mental illness, and medical condition. We expand on the setting of use to include the presence or absence of family, social supports, and community as well as the larger socioeconomic and cultural context and stressors. In this way, the nuances of each drug experience can be identified and traced to their source so that the right problems can be tackled in the right order.

In the Final Analysis . . .

What we're getting at here is that substance use is *not* simple. The disease theory has created a false dichotomy in which we either are or are not addicts. How people get involved and overinvolved with drugs cannot be limited to the brain and its imperial status in contemporary science and belief. Why you use drugs or alcohol is not simple. How you get in trouble is complicated. How you avoid trouble often depends on a number of variables in your life. *Harm reduction offers an infinitely flexible way of understanding your own problems with each drug that you use in your own context.*

What's Next?

In the next chapter, we will guide you through the model we use to establish your own understanding of each substance you use. In that process, you can analyze your unique relationship with each drug and begin to understand more precisely all of the factors contributing to your problems with drugs.

"Addiction" is not a disease—it is the result of a complicated interaction between your biology, psychology, and social situation.

You get to understand your relationship with drugs in the way that suits you best.

Many people mature out of drug problems—and you might be one of them!

5 How Do I Know If *I* Am in Trouble?

> *How much people drink may matter less than how they drink it.*
> —MALCOLM GLADWELL, *Drinking Games*

Gladwell is referring to culture. In his 2010 *New Yorker* article, he describes a discovery made by an anthropology student in the 1950s while doing research in Bolivia. In the village where he and his wife lived, very heavy drinking of very potent alcohol occurred every weekend. Yet despite the fact that most participants in the village's drinking rituals got drunk and passed out, there were no disputes and no aggression, only "pleasant conversation." When the couple returned to New Haven, Connecticut, they connected with the Yale University Center of Alcohol Studies. Their discovery coincided with research on the drinking patterns in the local Italian immigrant community where individuals drank every day, usually multiple times a day, yet had very low rates of alcoholism. The conclusion being drawn was that drinking problems have much more to do with culture than they do with alcohol.

As you go about trying to decide whether you are in trouble, pay close attention to the patterns—places, times, and activities—surrounding your use. Pay attention to which patterns are problems and which aren't. Are you or people around you suffering harm because of your drug use? Maybe you are; maybe you aren't. Maybe you are running into trouble with some of your drugs and not others. Maybe you are obnoxious or aggressive when you drink too much, but on meth you're energetic and witty, the life of the party. Maybe you use pills in dangerous ways that risk overdose, but marijuana is a mild high that makes you giggle at the wonder of it all. Whatever problems you are encountering, it is most likely that one factor didn't cause your problems. It's not the drugs. It's not you. It's not the environment. It's a unique combination of all three—a combination that is unique to you.

The previous chapter gave you several ways to think about your relationship with drugs—disease, learning, self-medication, trauma, and theories of vulnerability. In so doing, we offered you a menu of options that invites you to settle on a theory that best fits *your* relationship with drugs. We introduced you to the Drug, Set, Setting model, which can incorporate everything about you, your drugs, and the context in which you live and use drugs. Drug, Set, Setting allows you to tease out which aspects of different drugs are helpful and which are harmful. For example, you can use meth to get through a shift at the restaurant. It works, but probably contributes to exhaustion over time because you are working too hard, not getting enough rest, and overriding the need for rest by getting amped on speed. When you use meth at a sex party, on the other hand, any thought of condoms goes out the window. The risk of HIV, hepatitis, or other sexually transmitted diseases is 100 times more concerning than exhaustion. Pills (benzos or pain pills) can be used medicinally to manage anxiety or pain with great effect, but when used habitually to manage *life,* they become a problem. Pills won't solve your family problems, your employment problems, or your self-esteem issues. They will, however, provide some cushion against your *experience* of them. As long as the pills you buy are not of uncertain composition or dosage, they might be just the ticket to getting through a rough patch in your life.

In this chapter, you can use Drug, Set, Setting to lay out the details of your drug use so that you can see all sides of your relationship with drugs at once. You will be able to see which aspects have the greatest impact on the development of harm and which are most helpful. And it might well not be the drugs. It might instead be your disastrous marriage or the depression that has never responded well to treatment. It might be that you are getting high with people who love you, not that pot is the thing that soothes your soul. From there, you can consider which issues (if you decide you have issues) are most important for *you,* not your mother, your partner, or your therapist, to focus on first. By the end of this chapter you should have a pretty good idea where the trouble with drugs lies. Our hope is that Drug, Set, Setting will inform and empower you to prioritize what to start working on and what to leave for later.

When you dig into the details of your drugs, yourself, and your surroundings, remember that your drug use patterns have developed over time, so it might take some time to unravel it all. This can be overwhelming. Take it slow if you want. Think about yourself for as long as you can, then take a break!

Drug, Set, Setting: The Details

What do *drug, set,* and *setting* actually mean? What *are* they, and how do they impact your drug experiences and lead to problems? In this section, we will describe each in a fair amount of detail. Then we will illustrate how they interact by returning to Cheryl, Tyler, and Ruben.

Drug, Set, Setting provides a structure within which we can deconstruct the fine details of our drug use. It is like Monday-morning quarterbacking (a meme that is losing meaning as the pros now play several days a week). You wake up wondering why your team lost when they were doing so well. You review the plays of the day before and spot where the team went wrong. The quarterback chose the wrong play in the fourth quarter for his position on the field, and that was it. Or is it like analyzing a fight with your teenage daughter once it's over? You realize that the fight was not caused by the fact that she refused to agree to your curfew. It started way before that. She failed a math test; you, worried about paying for college, freaked out about her GPA ruining her chances of a scholarship. Her embarrassment intensified, and she rebelled at your (unnecessary) reminder that she be home on time.

Here is how it works with drugs:

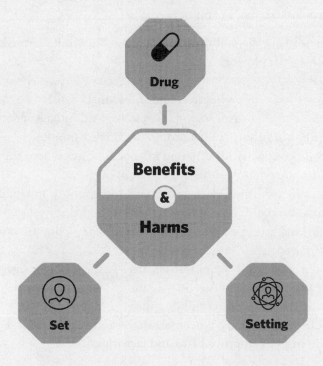

Drug

Each type of drug has its own unique chemistry and produces widely varied effects. How it is used changes its effects, as does how much and how often it is used.

What Kind of Drug

A drug's *action* is the first important element. Uppers, downers, all-arounders (also the name of an excellent guide to drugs by pharmacist Darryl Inaba)—these aren't technical terms, but you get the idea (a more detailed description of each drug is given in the quick reference at the back of this book). There are four broad types of drugs in terms of the *experience* they offer:

- **Stimulating** drugs—caffeine, cocaine, amphetamine-based drugs, nicotine, khat (cathinones), synthetic cathinones like bath salts

- **Sedating** drugs (central nervous system depressants)—opioids, benzodiazepines, or barbiturates, for example. Alcohol is a central nervous system depressant but at low doses can have a stimulating effect due to its disinhibiting properties.

- Drugs whose main effects are **perception altering**—hallucinogens, ecstasy, marijuana, ketamine

- **Disorienting or obliterating** drugs—PCP, inhalants like glue and gasoline, and poppers

This list is not comprehensive, and individuals can have markedly different reactions to each drug. Some people find marijuana sedating, others get silly, while still others get paranoid. Now, with hundreds of strains that are developed specifically for different effects, in states where this is possible we are able to buy what we want for different purposes.

Finally, and very important, drugs are increasingly not what they say they are. Pills, synthetic cannabinoids, heroin, and ecstasy are a crapshoot. Made in labs and factories all over the world, they contain multiple substances, many not fit for human consumption. Episodes of mass hospitalization are grabbing headlines as we write. If you are reading this in 10 years, there will be other

> Increasingly, drugs are not what they say they are.

headlines. Or drugs will have been legalized and regulated and your drugs will be made in FDA-approved labs and factories.

Route of Administration

How a drug is taken—*the route of administration*—influences how quickly and how dramatically the drug gets to your brain. There are four main routes of administration:

- **Smoking** is the fastest. The drug enters the bloodstream in the lungs and is immediately transported along with oxygen to the brain. The faster the drug comes on, the more compelling it is, which is one reason smoking crack became a larger problem than snorting cocaine ever was.

- **Injecting** into veins (IV) or into muscle (IM). IV is the most efficient way to get the greatest amount of the drug to your brain. Injecting into the muscle is not common except for ketamine (which is too hard to control by IV).

- **Snorting** or applying to other mucous membranes (booty bumping, for example).

- **Drinking or eating** is the slowest and least efficient method of absorbing drugs into the bloodstream because they don't enter the bloodstream until some of the drug has been processed (metabolized) by the digestive system and excreted. Alcohol is almost always ingested, or should be! Having said that, marijuana's effects are quite different, and desirable for many reasons, when eaten.

Dosage and Frequency

How *much* do you use, how *often,* and *when*? Small amounts may create euphoria. Larger amounts may cause "drunkenness" or overdose. Whether a drug is in its natural plant form, is the extracted active ingredient of the plant, or is made in a lab (synthetic) affects dosage: extracts or synthesized drugs are much more potent. A drug's legal status is very important. The quality control of illegal drugs is poor to nonexistent, making it hard to monitor dosage and impurities. Moreover, one often uses in a hurry to avoid being caught. Rushing your drug use can be dangerous, especially if you're injecting it and don't take the time to test a small amount for potency.

How often you use impacts your tolerance (ability to absorb the drug without having serious negative effects like overdose). If you are a maintenance user, you are likely dosing yourself on a regular schedule and thereby maintaining a steady state of intoxication—no dramatic ups and downs.

This does not necessarily protect you from overdose or other harms, but it does mean that you are more predictable. If you are a binger, you go on one- or several-day runs. Bingers tend to get blasted periodically and are pretty functional in between the parties or the solo three-day run. Judgment might be more impaired and drug-related risks more likely. Occasional use can be planned with care—a weekend in the mountains enhanced by psilocybin mushrooms or single-malt whiskey. Or it can be accidental

> Each use pattern works for some things, not for others.

and disastrous—a party that turned into a 2-day speed run.

When you use affects how well you manage your life. A bump of speed first thing can get you to that early-morning meeting. Smoking a bowl in the morning might be habitual, but it probably won't make you the star of the meeting! Of course, it depends on the meeting. Drinking in the evening is relaxing and fun, but at lunchtime your productivity suffers. Then there is using all day every day. At that point you are a maintenance user and perhaps a chaotic one. It has *become* your life.

Drug Combinations

Here are just a few major pointers. If you combine central nervous system depressants, you are at higher risk of overdose. Combining stimulants increases·your chances of heart attack or stroke. And if you mix sedating and stimulating drugs, one can mask the effects of the other, prompting you perhaps to take more to feel the effects. The details are important here, so refer to the quick reference section at the back of this book or to the references that we recommend elsewhere in the book.

Set

Set refers to you, the user, and aspects of yourself—your personality, your health, and your motivations—that interact in healthy and unhealthy ways with the drugs you use. *Set* originally referred mostly to your personality and your mind-set at the time of using. We use it more broadly to factor in all of who you are.

General Characteristics: Age, Gender, Race, Sexual Orientation, Ethnicity, Identity, Culture, and Socioeconomic Status

Older people tend to be more sensitive to the effects of drugs (and medications) and so need less to get the desired effect. Women have approximately

50% less of the stomach enzyme that metabolizes alcohol than men do, so women become more intoxicated at a lower dose. Approximately 50% of people in certain racial groups, primarily Asian, lack an enzyme in the liver that metabolizes alcohol. This causes "flushing" and headaches while drinking because your body is reacting to alcohol as a poison. Gender identity and sexual orientation are factors. Historically, substance misuse has occurred at far higher rates among gay and transgender people. Fear, rejection, danger, secrecy, and stigma are the likely causes.

Your *cultural identity* and the extent to which you feel identified and secure as a member of a group are important. Does your ethnic group or region of the country have particular attitudes toward drug use? Of course they do—does that create internal conflicts for you? Do you feel alienated from your culture of origin, either because you don't like its members or because they've rejected you? Have you taken on another identity about which you feel good? The most common examples are when young people (or adults, for that matter) come out as gay, get involved in an interracial relationship, or develop a radically different political orientation from their family or community of origin. Or choose to join a drug-using subculture. It is then that rejection and alienation can take a serious toll on self-esteem or create feelings of depression and anger.

We use the term *socioeconomic status* (or SES) because we are thinking particularly about money and other resources, but many people also like to be clear about the class to which they belong—working class, executive class, and so forth. Access to resources is an important contributor to harm. If you have little money and are buying on the streets, your risk of dirty drugs is greater. If, on the other hand, you have a lot of money to spend on a large stash, you can get closer to the source and buy purer drugs. Money also influences where you use and your access to clean water, privacy, and good food. A homeless injection drug user has much more to worry about than one who lives in a nice house.

Personality

Are you a risk taker? Do you love a challenge? This personality trait may make it easier for you to experiment with different drugs than it would be for someone who is a more cautious type. Are you naturally cautious or conservative? If so, you are more likely to plan carefully and avoid risky drug-taking situations. You are also more likely to use the first time with an experienced user. Do you want a new view or understanding of life? A search for meaning and insight may motivate you to try LSD or other hallucinogens. Are you a rebel? Do you think people in authority are frauds?

You might be more willing to use illegal drugs than is the person who has a deeper respect for authority. Do you want to hang out in groups and be close to people? Ecstasy might be the drug you choose.

Motivation for Using, Expectation of Effect, Mood at Time of Using

Your *mood,* what *motivates* you to use a drug, and what you *expect* from it influence the experience you have. People who use cannabis and hallucinogens like LSD probably know this. Your mood and your expectation influence how high you get, whether you get relaxed, silly, talkative, sleepy, or anxious, and whether you have a "good trip" or a "bad trip." This phenomenon has been studied with alcohol. When given nonalcoholic drinks that they are told contain alcohol, people show many of the same signs of intoxication as those who were actually given alcohol! In other words, what you expect to happen is more likely to happen. This is also true in "relapse." When people believe that "one drink leads to a thousand," a hopeless mind-set kicks in and makes it so—the abstinence violation effect, aka "What the hell!"

Health (Physical, Mental, and Emotional) and Medications

Do you have a medical condition that makes certain physical or organ systems more vulnerable, such as liver disease, high blood pressure, lung disease, or diabetes? Do you have a mental or emotional condition that makes you more susceptible to the effects of certain drugs? For example, are you normally anxious? Taking cocaine, a stimulant that activates norepinephrine, the fight–flight neurotransmitter, could make you paranoid. Are you taking medications that might interact with your chosen recreational drugs? If you aren't aware of any particular emotional vulnerability, you might get clues about what underlying or coexisting mental, physical, or emotional issues you have by noticing that you're drawn to a particular kind of drug (either depressants, stimulants, or consciousness-changing drugs).

Setting

Where you use and the larger environmental influences can be as important as who you are or what you use.

   Setting refers to the *environment* in which you drink or use drugs. This covers the culture of your using group and the social controls and using norms practiced by that group as well as the safety or danger of the place where you use. Who are you usually with, and where are you? Alone? With friends or family? Outside under a freeway overpass or inside a dry apartment with running water? The setting will determine not only what drug you might use but also the effect it will have on you. An important harm reduction fact discovered in recent years is that people overdose more easily on heroin when they use the same drug in an unfamiliar environment or when alone. Shooting heroin in a back alley is not as safe as shooting it at home. Home is usually cleaner, has running water, and, unless you have people there you're trying to hide from, you're not as rushed, so you can be careful to do it right. Where and with whom you use psychedelics such as LSD makes a very big difference in whether you have a "good trip" or a "bad trip." Drinking alone is a different experience from drinking with others. It could be anything from more depressing to more relaxing. Most important, if you're using a drug that is associated with lethal overdose or accidents—heroin, alcohol, ecstasy, nitrous, ketamine, or solvents, for example—using with others around who have the ability to take care of you in an emergency (if they aren't too loaded themselves or too afraid to call 911) could save your life.

The *larger context*—the attitudes and beliefs of your community and the dominant culture around you regarding drugs—and the *legal environment* surrounding each drug heavily influence the existence or absence of social controls and rituals that guide drug use. Many people define their community primarily by their personal relationships with their families and friends. But *community* can describe everything from your religious affiliation to your local political and social environment. What are some of the unique beliefs, traditions, and activities associated with your culture? Does religion play a big part? How about social activities? Do people in your culture spend most of their time with family, or are friends just as important? Is it expected that you marry and have children to fit in? What if you don't? How do people feel about celebration and fun? Is it part of how life is supposed to be lived, or is hard work more valued? On the one hand, these cultural forces have made you who you are. On the other, you may be alienated from your culture of origin. Perhaps you grew up in a strong Italian Catholic culture but now you're a lesbian, and women in that culture are supposed to get married and have children (with a man). Or perhaps you married young and raised a family, but now you want to travel and not be part of a multigenerational family. The conflicts you feel will certainly affect your tendency to use drugs or alcohol in a way that may be different from others in your family of origin. An interesting finding is that heavy opioid users in the United States suffered severe psychosocial consequences at a rate much higher than those in

Britain. The researchers thought that perhaps the more liberal beliefs among the British regarding drugs allowed drug users the psychological freedom to develop rituals and rules that helped contain their use and minimize abuse by using within their own social group.

The setting also refers to the *stresses* and the *supports* in your life. Do you have a job and enough money, or are you poor? Do you have family to take care of, or are you responsible only for yourself? What is the quality of your relationships with family members? Are you hiding your drug use from your spouse, kids, parents, or siblings? Are they aware of it and worried about you? Are they ashamed of you? And what about other relationships—do you have supportive friends or a group with whom you spend time? Do your friends encourage you in healthy or unhealthy choices and behaviors?

How Drug, Set, Setting Works

Cheryl, Tyler, and Ruben

Cheryl, Tyler, and Ruben all have unique characteristics and issues. In the Drug, Set, Setting diagrams on pages 97–99, look at how their issues get laid out.

Making the Connections

Lines can be drawn between specific use patterns and set and setting issues. The Drug, Set, Setting diagram illustrates all of the factors relevant to a person's drug use. Here is how we explain the relationship between the factors. With some of her drinking, Cheryl is trying to manage the stress of her job and of sexual intimacy. But she has hypertension, which can be exacerbated by excessive alcohol use. She also wants a relationship with a man but has a personal history that makes this difficult. While alcohol relaxes her enough to enable sex, it also unleashes anger that provokes fights. The effects of combining drugs are creeping up on her with a Vicodin habit that has outlived its medical usefulness. That puts her at risk of overdose, especially because she drinks so much when she is alone.

The possible relationships between personal, drug, and setting characteristics are numerous. When you develop your own Drug, Set, Setting matrix for each of your drugs, you can draw lines between any factors that seem to have an impact on each other. You don't need to worry too much about what *caused* what, although that is important too. The goal of this model is to help you figure out where to start. It is like unknitting a sweater.

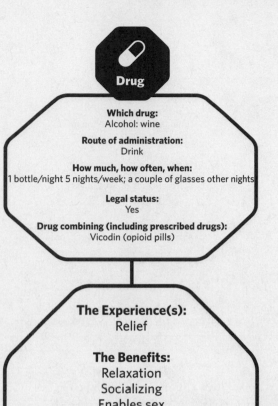

Drug

Which drug:
Alcohol: wine

Route of administration:
Drink

How much, how often, when:
1 bottle/night 5 nights/week; a couple of glasses other nights

Legal status:
Yes

Drug combining (including prescribed drugs):
Vicodin (opioid pills)

Cheryl

The Experience(s):
Relief

The Benefits:
Relaxation
Socializing
Enables sex

The Harms:
Fights
Hard to get up for work/exhausted
Combined with pills
Risk of overdose or falling

Set

General:
46-year-old African American heterosexual woman who grew up in middle-class family in a small southern town

Identity/affiliation/occupation:
Successful black professional (attorney); involved in many activities in community; community is other professionals

Personality type:
Friendly and kind but somewhat reserved; awkward in intimate relationships

Motivation for using/expectation of what will happen:
Relaxation; helps with sex; it always works

Health (physical, mental, emotional, medications):
Hypertension; PTSD from childhood sexual abuse; fatigue

Setting

Setting of use:
Home or out with friends; on dates

The larger community (accepting, alienating, dangerous?):
Friends are worried; hiding illegal pill use; family and larger community would be shocked

Life stresses:
High-stress job; relationships with men

Supports:
Good friends; well-regarded in her community; loving parents

Tyler

Drug

Which drug:
Stimulant: methamphetamine

Route of administration:
Smokes

How much, how often, when:
100 mg/day during the week;
0.5 gram/day on weekends

Legal status:
No

Drug combining (including prescribed drugs):
With alcohol (especially on weekends)

The Experience(s):
Life of the party
Effective at work

The Benefits:
Can party all night
Great concentration at work
(with small doses)
Decreases loneliness

The Harms:
Drinks more
Misses works some Mondays
Depressed after
heavy use

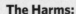

Set

General:
Late 20s white Jewish
heterosexual man raised
in middle-class family

Identity/affiliation/occupation:
Party animal, middle-income/class,
newspaper editorial job

Personality type:
Quiet, studious, hard working

**Motivation for using/expectation
of effect of what will happen:**
Fun, companionship, energy at work

**Health (physical, mental,
emotional, medications):**
Looking tired, lonely

Setting

Setting of use:
Club, bars, friends' houses

**The larger community
(accepting, alienating, dangerous?):**
Disapproving; his friendship circle is
starting to ease off their partying;
they are maturing out

Life stresses:
Absence of friends or activities
outside of partying;
no romantic relationships

Supports:
Some friends; mostly he drinks
and parties with them

Drug

Which drug:
Cannabis: marijuana

Route of administration:
Smokes

How much, how often, when:
4–5 bowls a day, throughout the day

Legal status:
Legal in California

Drug combining (including prescribed drugs):
Poppers, cocaine, ecstasy, alcohol

Ruben

The Experience(s):
Acceptance

The Benefits:
Relief from worry about HIV
Feels some moments of joy
Helps him forget traumatic memories

The Harms:
Sometimes anxious and paranoid
Trouble concentrating at work
Lung irritation

Set

General:
31-year-old Latino man
raised in a traditional Catholic
family in rural California;
second-generation American;
working class

Identity/affiliation/occupation:
Part of gay community; unstable work

Personality type:
Loving and gregarious

**Motivation for using/expectation
of what will happen:**
Numb out memories;
social belongingness

**Health (physical, mental,
emotional, medications):**
HIV; on medications that
aren't working; depression
and anxiety

Setting

Setting of use:
Bars; parties; home

**The larger community
(accepting, alienating, dangerous?):**
Within community heavy drinking
and drug use is normative;
outside community
is disapproving; family very strict

Life stresses:
HIV; financial debts
from prior unemployment

Supports:
Some friends, but minimal support
outside the gay community;
family cut him off because he
is gay, do not know he has HIV

If you don't want to take scissors to it and cut it into pieces (which means you have to throw away an entire sweater's worth of yarn), you have to find a piece of yarn that will start the process of unraveling. With Drug, Set, Setting you can grab the low-hanging fruit, the easiest thing to start with, and it will begin the process of change. But that is for the next few chapters. For now, it is time to diagram your own drug, set, and setting.

Now Your Drug, Set, Setting Diagram

You identified the reasons you use in Chapter 2 and began identifying the harms of your use in Chapter 3. Now you have a chance to see the interactions between your drug, set, and setting. Just as we demonstrated with Cheryl, Tyler, and Ruben, use the diagram on page 101 (or see the end of the Contents for information on printing out additional copies) to create your own Drug, Set, Setting diagram. Use one form for each drug—the relationships between each drug and your set and setting might be quite different. Then start drawing connections between drug, set, and setting factors. You can play with the connections for days or weeks. Drug, Set, Setting is a relational thought process that is radically different from the drug-focused hierarchy of the disease model. It takes time and practice to become fluent. We give you one diagram here. To make additional copies for each additional drug you use, photocopy the worksheet in this book or go to the website to print or fill in extras online (see the box at the end of the table of contents).

> Drug, Set, Setting is a relational thought process that is radically different from the drug-focused hierarchy of the disease model.

What Seems Most Important?

Before we end this chapter, it will be helpful if you highlight the issues that are causing you most concern. This will begin the process of prioritizing what you will work on first. And lest we have not said this enough, you might not start with the drugs!

What's Next?

You've done a lot of learning, thinking, feeling, and self-assessment up to now. You're probably thinking that it's time to get going, and fast. *But not*

My Drug, Set, Setting

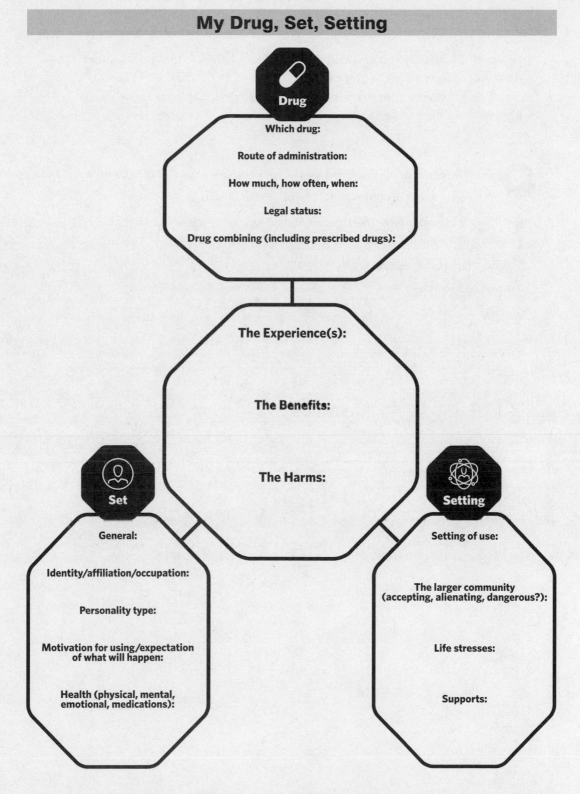

Drug

Which drug:

Route of administration:

How much, how often, when:

Legal status:

Drug combining (including prescribed drugs):

The Experience(s):

The Benefits:

The Harms:

Set

General:

Identity/affiliation/occupation:

Personality type:

Motivation for using/expectation of what will happen:

Health (physical, mental, emotional, medications):

Setting

Setting of use:

The larger community (accepting, alienating, dangerous?):

Life stresses:

Supports:

so fast. (Of course if you're doing things that are liable to kill you or others, then yes, change as fast as you can.)

The next section of the book will explain how people go about changing and help you make decisions and plans about the changes that *you* will make.

You are unique and complicated, and so is your drug use.

The social and legal context is as important as your drugs are to the quality of your drug experiences—both the benefits and the harms.

Sometimes the biggest problem is not the drugs!

6 How People Change

> *Habit is habit, and not to be flung out*
> *of the window by any man, but coaxed*
> *downstairs a step at a time.*
> —MARK TWAIN, *Pudd'nhead Wilson*

Habits are patterns that are ingrained in us. *Ingrained* means embedded, firmly fixed, and difficult to get rid of, like a red wine stain on your new white shirt. In other words, habits are hard to change because they have become part of how we live, just as the red wine molecules have become part of your shirt. Some of us hate change, some adapt begrudgingly, and some love change and embrace it with vigor. (Maybe the latter simply do not develop habits but bounce happily from one new activity to the next.) As we write this book, we are living in a culture that seems to value change over constancy. A dozen new smartphones every year, restaurants opening and closing by the minute, the latest fashions and endless apps—everything *new* is equated to progress.

> We worship all things new and seem to lack patience with and respect for the struggle to change ingrained habits.

It may not be surprising, then, that as a society we show little patience with or respect for how people actually struggle with changing deeply ingrained habits. When it comes to health-related behaviors, we all have difficulty with the time and energy that it takes to change. Getting a diagnosis of type 2 diabetes is a prime example. Typically people hear that news with a great deal of fear and vow to change their lifestyle fast: exercising more, losing weight, changing their diet, and checking their blood glucose levels throughout the day. We start strong. We get the ice cream out of the freezer, the cookies out of the cupboards, and vow to cook fresh food instead of heading for the drive-through after work. But after a few days or weeks most people slack off. You don't actually *have* time to shop and cook, the kids go nuts when they can't find the cookies, and you give in. Exercise is hard too. For "weekend warriors" that spurt of activity is more likely to result in pulled muscles than in the start of a new life that includes regular exercise. We cringe at the judgments we hear from our friends when they see us eating french fries.

Changing drug use is no different. While some people have an "aha" moment and seem to slide effortlessly into a new relationship with drugs (emphasis on *seem*), most of us change more slowly. "Just Say No" is a simple, powerful, and inspiring meme. The problem is, it is not how most people change.

This chapter is about how people change—about the change *process*. The research shows that most of us change incrementally; we take very tiny steps as we pass through several stages in our efforts to make lasting changes. We know from smoking cessation research that it takes an average of 7–10 attempts to quit for good. Among the people who quit taking drugs are those who quit the first time, but the people who seek harm reduction tend to be people who are struggling with change, or at least struggling with the limited options offered by traditional ways of thinking about drug use and misuse.

Harm reduction offers a wide variety of options for change and invites you to pick and choose *what* you address and *when*. In this chapter, we introduce you to a model of change, as well as some tools that have developed out of very robust research on motivation and change. Just sit back and read. You do not have to *do* anything except perhaps reflect on the concerns you highlighted in the last chapter. But only if you want to. Feel free to stand on Mark Twain's upstairs landing just as long as you need to and make sure your footing is secure as you proceed—no matter how slowly that is.

Before You Start

Not all change is arduous; you might find yourself doing something different rather effortlessly, sometimes without even thinking about it. We change all the time, in big or little ways. We start walking to the train station, stop nagging our partner about cleaning the kitchen, start flossing every night, or switch from whiskey to beer. In the substance use field, *maturing out, natural recovery,* and *spontaneous recovery* are terms used to describe the fact that most people who have problems with alcohol and other drugs resolve them on their own. Just think about all the people who have quit smoking, perhaps even yourself. Nicotine patches and counseling are very recent phenomena. Millions of people have quit, and most of them with no outside assistance. The same is true for most people who moderate or abstain from other drugs.

Why People *Don't* Change . . .

Being opposed to change supports the notion that you're just fine as you are. And why wouldn't you feel this way? After all, you've gotten this far, and you're still alive. Change is disruptive and implies a rejection of what *is* for what *might be*. Even though there are problems, it is sometimes easier and less painful to stick with the status quo than to risk what change *might* bring.

> In the words of economist John Kenneth Galbraith, "Given a choice between changing and proving that it is not necessary, most of us get busy with the proof."

Resistance

We vote with our feet. This is one way to recognize resistance. If we don't like something, we leave or we don't show up in the first place. Basically, we go on strike, especially if we have been told we *have* to study harder, quit smoking, or lose 10 pounds. If someone has said to you "Do something about your drinking" or "Spend more time with me" or "If you don't quit soon, you're going to ruin your life," what do you do? You cancel the next dinner with the person, forget to call her back, miss the next appointment, use more drugs. This is called *resistance.* When we are told to do something, most of us resist. We react against other people's scolding and warnings. Even when there's no outside pressure, even when we *want* to do something different, most people are allergic to change. We break out in a rash of resistance and fear.

This is completely normal, but why?

1. We just can't quite believe it's really that bad.
2. Resistance is powerful. After all, it is the source of social justice movements—from civil rights to animal protection and environmental rights. Resistance is the source of both freedoms and protections.
3. Better the devil we know than the one we don't. This adage is supported by the science of *homeostasis,* the law of inertia. As mammals, we cannot tolerate dramatic changes in our body temperature. We go into shock or die. Our psychology seems to follow this need to stay within a narrow comfort range. Change suggests going from the known to the unknown and losing something in the process.

Despite our tendency to resist, most people would, in fact, like to change *something* related to their drug use. If you could get rid of the hangover after a night at the bar, life would be great—no problems concentrating at work and no suspicious glances from your colleagues. If you could afford a babysitter so you and your partner could stay out late *together,* then no more nagging. If you could control your meth smoking so you could maximize the euphoria and avoid the paranoia that follows, you'd be happy. These situations illuminate the wish to change *at least something,* a wish that might remain hidden if you're surrounded by people who say you have to quit. (Note that all of these changes would be helpful and none require you to quit.)

Ambivalence

The word that best describes how most of us feel about change is *ambivalence.* Ambivalence means having mixed feelings about something, being "on the fence." On the one hand, I'm proud that my children made it to adulthood, but on the other I'll miss them terribly. I love my new apartment and the extra rooms that I'll have to set up an office and have guests, but it'll never be the same as the one where I spent my first 10 years out of school. I need to stop drinking—I don't have the energy I did in my 20s and 30s—but I'm not sure I can leave it behind; after all, it helped me cope for 10 years with the worst boss I've ever had.

Change is a good thing that has cured cancers and put 28 varieties of breakfast cereal on the grocery store shelf. Change has helped difficult marriages become easier ones and sad children become happy ones. But our "just do it" society makes very little room for the human experience of ambivalence. "Just do it" means we are expected to go from thinking to action in a nanosecond. "Just do it" suggests that even if there are obstacles, we should

> Our "just do it" society leaves little room for ambivalence.

"get over it" and move on. Or "get on with it" and open a new chapter in our life. We see this in how little time we allow people to grieve major losses. While the grief process takes years, we tend to stop asking people about their losses after a couple of months.

And while ambivalence is the hallmark of contemplating new things, we don't necessarily stop being ambivalent after we've moved on. You might not eat bacon for breakfast anymore, but you're still wishing you could!

Harm reduction puts the human experience of ambivalence ("I'm not sure if I want to or *can* just do it") at the center of its philosophy and invites you to respect and embrace both sides of your relationship with drugs. Ambivalence is the single most important feeling to pay attention to in practicing harm reduction. It means giving equal weight to the "yes" and the "but" of change. "Yes, but" is often seen as making excuses to keep using when really what's happening is that you're considering both sides. As you come to accept how drugs are harming you, also appreciate that you love them, or you did at one time. Deny-ing that love will have you sneaking around behind your own back to keep stoking the embers of a relationship you promised to extinguish forever.

> Harm reduction puts the human experience of ambivalence ("I'm not sure if I want to or *can* just do it") at the center of its philosophy and invites you to respect and embrace both sides of your relationship with drugs.

Honesty is needed to admit to yourself that change might be needed, but tremendous honesty is required to think of all the reasons *not* to change. It runs counter to our dominant culture of action. But the stronger the pull in either direction, the deeper the ambivalence. Ambivalence doesn't mean you're stuck. It doesn't mean you're in denial. It means you're waking up to the different directions in which you're feeling pulled. The more conscious you are of your ambivalence, the more realistic you will be in the promises you make and the more likely you will be to keep them.

Effort

While researching reasons that people give for continuing to try to make changes, Janet Polivy and Peter Herman realized that there are three main reasons people fail to make changes despite their desire to do so:

1. We underestimate how much effort will be required to make the change.
2. We underestimate how long we'll have to make the effort.
3. And we often *overestimate* the benefits of making the change.

The first two make sense. We hit a wall when we realize how *hard* it is! But the last reason is puzzling. Of course there are benefits—that's why we decided to change in the first place! We had really good reasons. But we might have had expectations that just didn't materialize. If I decide to lose weight for health reasons and lose 25 pounds yet find that my cholesterol and blood pressure are *still* too high, it just sucks. Or I might decide to stop smoking weed because my memory is not very good, only to find that now I'm having trouble sleeping—*and* my memory still isn't that great.

Big changes may be wonderful, but they may also not result in the won-derful things you imagined. So to make changes that you can stick with, you'll have to revisit your hopes, your expectations, and your motivations many times to make sure they are realistic and achievable.

. . . And How People *Do* Change

Motivation

Motivation is a basic ingredient in the willingness and ability to make changes. Motivation involves having energy, a sense of direction, and the persistence to accomplish things. Some motivation is *intrinsic*. We are internally driven to *do* something. Little effort is involved, and the sensation or activity—eating good food, playing with our toys, having sex, talking with friends—is usually pleasurable. Other motivation is *extrinsic*. This means being pushed to do something by outside forces, sometimes with the promise of rewards or threats of punishment. It involves doing things that are valued by others but may or may not be rewarding in themselves (cleaning the house, getting on the treadmill, doing homework, or going to work, for example). In general, changes that are driven by outside pressure tend to make it harder to make and maintain changes. When we do something because we *want* to (intrinsic), we feel more confident and powerful, our self-esteem goes up, and so does our sense of well-being. In turn, we gain the ability to regulate feelings and control impulses. When we do something that is motivated by outside forces, the opposite happens—unless we can take in (not resist) and integrate that outside motivation and make it our own.

How do we get from unwillingness to engagement, from extrinsic to intrinsic motivation? In other words, how does "I *should* change" become "I *want* to change"?

> According to Bill Miller, whose life work is developing ways to help people change, "Everyone is motivated for *something*. Our job is to help people figure out what the *something* is."

Self-Determination

Researchers Richard Ryan and Edward Deci have done extensive research on motivation and have found that the key to increasing motivation is *self-determination*. They identified three ingredients of intrinsic motivation. The same three ingredients help us internalize and integrate extrinsic motivation:

1. *Support and reinforcement from significant others*: When we experience empathy, curiosity, and support from those we admire, we are motivated to go along with them. Sometimes literally—to follow in their footsteps.

2. *A sense of competence*: The feeling that *I can do this* is highly motivating. Who doesn't want to do more of what he or she is good at? It feels good. A sense of competence is the same as self-efficacy, the belief that one can be effective in accomplishing a particular thing.

3. *A sense of autonomy*: This feeling that "I am the author of my own actions" is fostered by having choices and by having the respect of others to make those choices. Autonomy does not mean independence. One can be autonomous in an interdependent world. It simply means having some control, even if that is shared with others.

What gets in the way of developing intrinsic motivation? Not surprisingly, it's the opposite of the three factors that help us develop internalized motivation:

1. External control: coercion and mandates
2. Alienation: being rejected and isolated
3. Rewards and punishments

Navigating the Stages of Change

Change is not a threshold that you step over. It is true that some people wake up one day and, as if struck by a bolt of lightning, decide "I am going to move to New York" or "I no longer want to be married to my husband" or "I am going to quit my Wall Street job and be the artist that I was in my 20s" or "I'm done with cigarettes. I'm quitting." Most of us, however, don't change that easily.

Nor is harm reduction a "hit bottom and surrender" model. We do not subscribe to the notion that people need to bottom out before they find their way to "recovery." We have seen too many people who hit bottom and get stuck there. They go on until they have nothing left to lose, they adapt, and they accrue more and more obstacles to living a life free of trouble. They become homeless, hungry, and hopeless. Or they die along the way. This is not only entirely unnecessary but dangerous, and to prescribe bottoming out to anyone is, in our view, inhumane.

> Change is not a threshold that you step over. Nor is harm reduction a "hit bottom and surrender" model.

Instead, harm reduction meets people at *their* stage of change. The stages of change model was developed by psychologists James Prochaska and Carlo DiClemente. In their decades of research, they identified six stages that make up the process of change: pre-contemplation, contemplation, preparation, action, maintenance, and relapse (also called recycling). At some point, we are done and leave the process behind. We are over it. This stage is called termination. Each stage involves putting effort into somewhat different things in order to move along. Below is what it looks like.

Precontemplation

The *precontemplation* stage is the "Who, me?" stage. You wonder who they're talking about when they say you have a drinking problem. People give you a ton of information that you might accept or reject. Either way, you don't know what to do with these suggestions, warnings, ultimatums—except

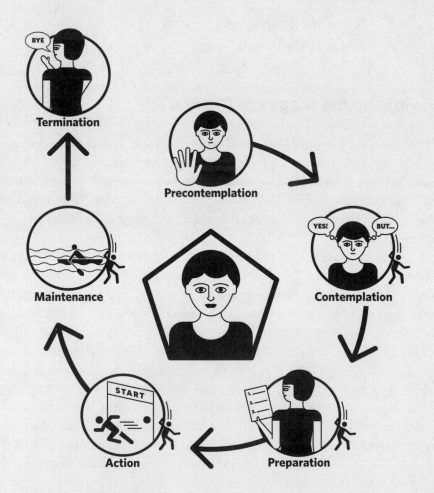

feel pangs of irritation or resentment before you pick up the glass or the pipe again. This is the stage at which many people think you are "in denial." But you are not denying anything; you just don't see what the people around you see. You feel badgered, and you stop listening.

Contemplation

Something happens, and often it's not good. You get a DUI, you get diagnosed with hepatitis C, you get a bad dose of ecstasy, you are inattentive at work and your colleagues start wondering about you. You start to worry. Alternatively, someone offers you solid information about the dangers of your substance use in a respectful enough manner that you listen. Either way, you start questioning your relationship with drugs. A third possibility is that you have arrived at a "maturing out" point in your life. You are growing up, taking on more responsibility in your work, committing to a relationship, or deciding to have children. You no longer want to maintain the party life or the late nights out with your wife. It's time to consider change.

The *contemplation* stage is the "Yes, but" stage. This is when you become torn between "on the one hand" and "on the other hand." In other words, you are ambivalent. As we said before, *ambivalence—being of two minds about something—is a perfectly normal part of change.* On the one hand, nothing takes you out of your boredom like a few hits of crack. On the other, you aren't doing well at work, and your boss is noticing. You're attracted to books that educate you, maybe even read a few that make you think about your use. Maybe you start talking to someone or check out a self-help meeting. You begin considering what making changes might look like. You begin to consider what choices you have.

The first time one of us (Jeannie) taught this model to a group of social service staff, some of whom were in abstinence-based recovery, one of the men began sobbing and said, "All these years I thought I was crazy. I hated myself for not 'getting it.' But really I was just in contemplation."

Preparation: Getting Ready

At some point, after weeks or months or years, you make a decision to *do* something. But action is *still* not usually your next move. Although there's nothing wrong with just going ahead and doing something, you don't want to just jump in and fail at what you do and get frustrated at yourself. Generally, people move into the *preparation* or the "Uh-oh" stage. The rubber begins to hit the road as you zero in on what to do. You might have decided not to smoke pot when you're taking care of your kids or not to share needles. But *how* should you follow through on this decision? If pot's in the house, you could roll a joint even in your sleep. And you haven't a clue where to get a large supply of needles. You explore ways to make your decision happen. Still, you're scared it won't help or you're just not up to it. If that happens, you should consider any other areas you could take care of first—perhaps getting treatment for depression, moving to a different neighborhood, hanging out with different friends. In addition you might begin to visualize a life that's different from the one you've lived up to now. This fantasy makes you feel jazzed about taking action, and you map out realistic plans for the action stage. You find out where the needle exchange program is in your community. You plan to store your pot at someone else's house and just get a limited supply every day.

Action: Ready, Steady, GO!

Finally, the "do it" stage. In traditional addiction models, "getting on with it," "just doing it," means quitting drugs. But in harm reduction, even the action stage is a bit more complex and allows for many different decisions about what and how much to change. In our model, in the action stage you've made a plan that includes a series of steps that are just the right size, and now you're taking those "right-sized steps," continually evaluating how it's going. Sometimes you feel like you can conquer anything. For example, you may quit drinking altogether. Or you stop injecting heroin and snort it instead. Whatever action you take, you try to take steps that won't be so big you trip on them.

Maintenance

The *maintenance* stage is "the grind." You're solidifying your progress, using support to work through underlying psychological troubles, and getting used to your new routines. Your sense of unfamiliarity and risk begins to fade. The world is not such a scary place, but it can be pretty tedious. Despite your exhilaration at times, every day you might feel like you're having your teeth extracted, and every minute the world feels like a scary place. There are times when you're bored out of your brain and pissed off that so much work is involved. This is a time when you might decide that you need therapy to deal with the loneliness, anxiety, or depression that has plagued you for years. Or you make some new friends who will support your efforts to stick with your changes. You change your environment to support your new behavior—a new job, a new friend. This might be when you realize you may need some antidepressant medication to help you stay on course. It might be that you take up playing the guitar to keep your hands busy or go back to your neighborhood church for a sense of community.

Recycling (Relapse)

When you don't seem to be progressing, or you slip back into the mind-set of a previous stage, you are recycling, more traditionally called a "relapse" or "setback." Sometimes what happens feels a little more like a bullet ricocheting! Relapse is not actually a stage. It simply means taking a step or two back, and this can happen at any point. In *relapse* you head "back to the drawing board." Relapse simply means breaking a promise you made to yourself or to someone else. It may be just a momentary lapse. It does not necessarily mean a return to using or using in the way you did before. It means looking at how the promise you made to yourself was unrealistic because you didn't take something into account.

You promised yourself that you wouldn't drink during the week, and it has worked pretty well for months. But your cousin's wedding was on a Wednesday evening, and they had an open bar, and you just hadn't planned on that. Or you had promised yourself you would use only clean needles but found yourself with a group of people who hadn't brought their own, and you ended up sharing. You smoked crack the day you learned your wife had a miscarriage. *Relapse often happens when you find yourself in a "high-risk" situation, without a specific plan.* Many of the harms that led you to action have been forgotten, but you can clearly remember the benefits of your favorite drug.

> Relapse simply means breaking a promise you made to yourself or to someone else.

You might also develop an "Oh, to hell with it" feeling after breaking your promise and be tempted just to trash the whole thing. Then you beat yourself up for your failure. But relapsing doesn't mean you didn't work hard enough. It means the plan was flawed or not complete enough to take into account all possible pitfalls—given the complexity of human life, what plan could possibly anticipate everything? You're allowed to go back to work on it. In doing so, you explore what worked and what didn't work. Congratulate yourself for your success. Feel as little shame as possible. Take it for what it was—a bump in the road. Move on and reevaluate your plan so that the next bump won't trip you up.

Termination

Termination is when you say "I'm over it." The work is done; you've ceased doing the harm you originally sought to reduce. It's at this point that you begin to recognize that your harmful relationship with drugs and/or alcohol is resolved. The difference between termination and precontemplation is that true awareness, or consciousness, has taken the place of your lack of knowledge and understanding of your experiences. You're harm-free, but not necessarily drug-free. You may have found a way to continue your use, but in a way that is controlled and healthier.

The next chapter will help you determine what stage of change you might be in and what is motivating you. But for now, there is another way to look at change.

> The difference between termination and precontemplation is that true awareness, or consciousness, has taken the place of your lack of knowledge and understanding of your experiences.

Readiness

The researchers who continually study motivation and develop motivational counseling (motivational interviewing) have opted to simplify the stages of change into levels of readiness. They have found that change is so fluid that it works better to simply identify where you are on the Readiness Ruler (see the drawing below). On any given day, or in any given week, you can slide

Are you not prepared to change, already changing, or somewhere in the middle?

0 1 2	3 4 5 6	7 8 9 10
Not ready	**Getting ready**	**Ready**

Not prepared   **Already changing**

back and forth between greater and lesser degrees of readiness. You can plot your progress using the Readiness Ruler as a simple tool. All of the factors that we have discussed so far—embracing and understanding your ambivalence, motivation, supportive relationships, self-efficacy, and autonomy—influence how ready you are to change.

The Language of Change

You can easily figure out how ready you are to change by paying attention to the language you use when you think about or talk about your problems. Researchers and counselors who specialize in motivation and change have identified two kinds of change language: *change talk* and *sustain talk*.

Change talk expresses our need, reasons, desires, ability, and commitment to change.

- *Need*: "I have to quit smoking" or "If I don't stop partying, I'll lose my job."

- *Reasons*: "If I socialized more, I'd feel less lonely."

- *Desire*: "I want to reduce my spending" or "I'd like to cut down on my speed use."

- *Ability*: "I know I can change my diet" or "I've got what it takes to quit heroin."

- *Commitment*: "I am going to start being nicer to myself" or "I've begun to cut back on my drinking."

Sustain talk refers to sustaining the status quo, maintaining things the way they are. These are things you say to others or to yourself that reflect your disbelief or your doubts that you should, that you want to, or that you *can* change.

- *Stay the same*: "If I didn't have my private time, I'd go crazy," "I need my pain pills," "If I drank less, I would be more tense," or "I can't quit smoking; it's too hard."

How Cheryl Is Talking

Cheryl hasn't done anything yet about her drinking or her pill use, but that doesn't mean she isn't having private, internal conversations. Some of the language she is using reflects both her desire to change and her resistance.

Change talk:

"I know I'm drinking too much, and I want to get a handle on it."

"It's not really helping me at work, and it's making my relationships worse."

"It shouldn't be too hard. I didn't used to drink this much."

"I'm worried about my use of pills."

"I need to make a plan to quit using pills."

Sustain talk:

"I won't be able to relax without wine."

"Drinking is the only way I can enjoy sex."

"It's not really that much compared to other people I know."

"I get shaky when I try not to take the pills."

"Maybe I could just use them till I get my stress under control."

For now, these conversations don't seem to be helping her make changes. But she is identifying both her motivations and her resistances. It will take more conversations like this to help her move through the stages of change

Remember: we're not just saying what we already know when we talk this way; we're actually discovering our own attitudes and wishes as we listen to ourselves. You can hear your own ambivalence by paying attention to how you talk. The words you use correlate pretty well with what stage of change you are in. Change and sustain talk, as well as your level of ambivalence, can help identify your level of readiness. "I can't," "don't know how," or "don't know what I'd do" indicate lower levels of readiness. "I have to," "want to," and "know I can" signal higher levels of readiness. Keep this in mind as you prepare for the next chapter. If you want to, but *only* if you want to, you can reflect on the concerns you identified in the last chapter to see what you are saying to yourself.

What's Next?

In this chapter we've offered you a menu of options, knowing that we all have our preferred ways of thinking. The stages of change, the Readiness

Ruler, and the language of change are three different models that can help you conceptualize your process of change. Any of the three, or all of them together, can be the foundation for your next steps. Choose whatever works best for you.

In the next chapter we will help you develop your change plan. If you're not ready, just put the book down, or flip to the quick reference section that talks about how drugs work and study the drugs you use.

Respect your ambivalence—it is normal and necessary.

Everyone is motivated for *something,* and so are you.

Change is a process, not a threshold you step over.

7 You Don't Have to Quit to Change

The more things change, the more they stay the same.
—Jean-Baptiste Alphonse Karr,
French novelist and horticulturist

This seemingly paradoxical proverb means different things to different people. To us, it captures the reality that the more dramatic the change, the more intense the resistance and the more fiercely we cling to the status quo. Fortunately, you don't have to—and, in fact, can't—do everything at once.

Before You Start

Just because something is a problem doesn't mean you have to do something about it. We all have problems that we just live with. Because harm reduction is about options, you can pick and choose what you address and when.

"Start where the client is" is the first principle of harm reduction. As you read this book, you are both counselor and client. So pay close attention to where you are, not where someone (including you!) thinks you ought to be.

Change means loss. Getting thin means losing weight, perhaps weight we have had around since childhood, weight that has served as both burden and protector. Our children's growing up means losing them from our day-to-day lives. Moving to a great new place means leaving the last one, with all the experiences we had there. Getting a new job means leaving the one where we felt so competent, even if we hated the boss or the politics. And where drugs or alcohol are concerned, we have always thought change meant quitting—losing the medicine that has gotten us through so many hard times or losing the magic potion that has given us our most intense highs.

Choose right-sized steps. To avoid the ricochet effect, one must avoid overshooting in the first place.

Success breeds success. We recommend that you start with the issues that you are readiest to change. The reason is simple—you will meet less internal resistance and therefore be more likely to succeed. Success builds self-efficacy—a sense that you are *capable,* that you *can.* And self-efficacy leads to higher levels of motivation.

Change is a process, not an event.

Zeroing In on Your Alcohol and Drug Use

In this chapter we take you through your own change process, beginning with the crucial decision about whether or not to change anything. We will focus primarily on what you want to change about your substance use. First, we ask you to make a "wish list" of what you would like to change and what your goal is for each of your drugs. You will evaluate your readiness to tackle each issue. Then you'll use the stages of change to figure out the work that you need to do to accomplish each goal. Finally, we introduce you to a tool for working on the issues that you are still ambivalent about. The goal of this chapter is to help you prioritize the problems you have identified and set goals.

In Chapter 5 you highlighted *all* the aspects of your drugs, yourself (set), and your setting that concern you. You probably identified many concerns other than drugs—depression, anxiety, relationship, children, job stress, things that are tied up with and perhaps drive your drug use. As we guide you through a change process with drugs, your set and setting issues will show up in some of the steps you will need to take to change your relationship with drugs. You might decide, for example, that until you change your job, there's no way you can change your speed use. Or you might realize that your relationship keeps you in a state of uneasiness or fear. If so, you can put your drinking on the back burner for now. The tools that follow can be used to plan the steps for working on any and all of your issues.

The Choices

To Change . . .

If you find yourself faced with the dilemma of doing something about your relationship with drugs, you have choices about how to proceed. In all simplicity, in no particular order, and with absolutely no sarcasm, they are:

1. Change.
2. Don't change.

Change can mean changing everything, like discontinuing all use of all drugs. Or it can mean changing only some things, like limiting when you use or how much. It can mean changing how you use, like switching from needles to snorting. For example:

Change everything. Abstain from using all drugs. Do this all at once ("cold turkey"), with the help of others—a program or a therapist or friends—or on your own. Or warm turkey—cut down on one drug at a time, until you've eliminated it from your life. Or cut down on all of them simultaneously by tapering at a pace that you choose. Try periods of abstinence just to see what it feels like. Or moderate your use of everything or quit some and moderate others. You'll lower your tolerance this way, so you don't have to use as much to get a buzz when you start again—it's a tapering device.

Eliminate one drug and keep the others. Eliminate the most harmful one and don't do a thing about the others. Many people quit heroin but continue to drink or smoke meth. Another common change is to quit meth but keep drinking. You can eliminate the most harmful drug quickly or slowly and with or without assistance—it doesn't matter as long as it works for you.

A variation on the theme: eliminate more than one of the most harmful drugs and keep the rest. You might stop snorting cocaine because it's draining your bank account *and* quit drinking because you have hepatitis C, but keep your pot and enjoy ecstasy or ketamine from time to time.

Another variation: switch from more harmful to less harmful drugs. If you're clear that you aren't ready for, or interested in, a drug-free life, consider marijuana instead of heroin or pills. Or, if your drug use is driven by anxiety, see if you can find a doctor who understands that there are valuable antianxiety medications that are not used addictively by most people, including those who have a history of addiction. Or try an SSRI like fluoxetine (Prozac) or citalopram (Celexa).

Change how you use and with whom. Change the route of administration—snort instead of shoot so you eliminate the harm of needle use. Mix your scotch with water and ice so the first drink doesn't hit you so hard and cloud your judgment about whether to have another. Stop using alone so you won't die if you overdose—have someone there to call 911 or do rescue breathing.

Change how often or when you use. Stop using before work. Don't drink during the week, or at least not every night. Give your body a break. Smoke after the kids are in bed or only when you're out of the house.

In short, changing means taking control of *whatever* you can *whenever* you can. Whatever our society says, these are all legitimate options! It's all progress, and progress is success. It doesn't have to be all or nothing to be better. As our colleague Ken Anderson from HAMS says, "Better is better." Remember, **any positive change**.

. . . Or Not to Change

Although we've specifically mentioned this point earlier, it deserves to be repeated. No change, in traditional "addiction" circles, is a deal breaker. It is the one choice that will almost certainly get you excluded from any treatment or support network. The traditional thinking is that once you have decided not to make any changes, you're resistant, not ready, unmotivated. Your best bet is to go away until you bottom out—until you "get it."

But not changing your drug use doesn't mean you're doing nothing. It can mean doing more research. It can mean talking to someone about your problems. It can mean sitting with your fears and your mixed feelings and getting to know them better as you continue to use. It can mean doing absolutely nothing except noticing you've made a choice to do nothing. Changing can also mean returning to an activity that was positive for you—reading, walking, basketball, knitting. It doesn't always have to be something new or scary. And it doesn't have to be about drugs.

> Not changing your drug use doesn't mean you're doing nothing.

You could do many things while not changing your drug use:

- *Accept yourself as a drug user and embrace your ambivalence about change.*

- *Find people who accept you as a drug user.* Avoid judgmental people. Or work on them to stop ragging you about your relationship with drugs.

- *Educate yourself about safer drug use.* Learn overdose prevention and proper injection techniques. Don't let others shoot you up. Use clean syringes. Don't share pipes or come with your own mouthpiece. Make sure your ecstasy is really E. Use hallucinogens in a planned way and in the right setting for you. Don't let anyone else give you a drug you don't know about. Have a rule that you'll use a "designated driver" even if you have to use a paid designated driver to get you home.

- *Pay attention to yourself on drugs.* This is hard, especially if your goal is to get wasted, party hard, or obliterate painful feelings. But notice what you can. How impulsive are you when you're high on speed, and what tricks can you use to have safer sex? What are you like when you drink, or what do people tell you about your behavior if you drink yourself into a blackout? Do you fall down a lot when you use ketamine? Just notice these things, or try to accept others' observations, to build an accurate picture of yourself on drugs.

• *Ponder what you use drugs for.* You might already know a lot about why you use, things about your history, your discomfort with your life, or your desires for joy and new perspectives that make drugs compelling. As you use, get specific about what precise experience you are looking for with each drug. What do you feel after two drinks, and is it what you wanted to feel before you started? Then how do you feel after four, five, or six? What does pot do for you, and how many hits does it take to do it? Observe how you feel at different levels of use. You might even jot some of these observations down in a journal *while you're using* and read them later.

• *Do other things to be a healthy and balanced person.* Eat. Drink water. Stay warm. Exercise. Just a little. Look at something pretty every day. Talk to somebody nice. If you don't know anyone nice, go to a friendly store and buy a soda, just to talk to the cashier for a minute.

• *Use within your means, both financial and emotional.* You don't have to quit to keep some money in your pocket, your house, your job, your family, your friends, or your spirit.

Since change involves making conscious choices, the choice *not* to change should be equally conscious. If you have weighed all the options, and you decide to quit thinking, *you have still engaged in a positive process that has already changed you.* Despite the fact that no apparent change has been made,

> A start is more than you had yesterday.

you are still on the road. It may not result in an obvious reduction of harm, but it is a start, and a start is more than you had yesterday. *That's harm reduction.*

The Options:
Safety, Control, Moderation, and Abstinence

In Chapter 6 we explained *how* people change and gave you tools that you can use to manage your change process. Now you come to the task of deciding *what* to do next. Here are the options, laid out as simply as possible. Just as your drugs (or other issues) can step up from nonproblematic to chaotic, they can step down to safety, control, moderation, or abstinence.

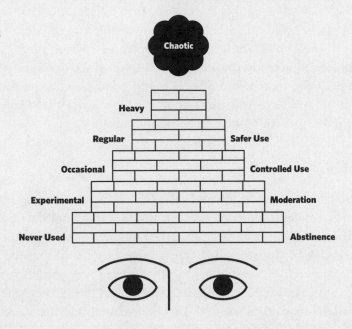

Safety

Safety means taking care. It might not mean changing anything about what or how much you use. It means not getting high and driving. It means shooting clean—using a new syringe each time you inject. It means using opioids with people who can administer naloxone or call 911 if you overdose. It means not sharing a crack pipe or bringing your own tip. It means not getting drunk or high around people that you care about if you tend to get abusive. It means avoiding the worst consequences of intoxication—the risk of serious harm to yourself and other people. Once you have established *safety,* you can put energy into thinking about *cutting back* or *quitting.*

> Safety first; then you can put energy into thinking about cutting back or quitting.

Control

Closely related to safety, control means developing a set of rules that you can use to "box yourself in" to safer and more conscious use. It is not necessarily about using less or none at all, although it can be. *Know* how high you want to get and limit the money in your pocket to the necessary amount. (And leave your bank card at home.) Keep your drugs in a place that requires effort to get to so that you have to be intentional when you use. Decide firmly when and where you will get high to reduce the temptation to give in to any offer or craving. Avoid situations or people that have caused you harm in the past. Any of these rules can help you feel more in control, more powerful, and more able to actually think about what you want to experience from your drugs. *If* you want to cut down or quit, controlling is the first step in that direction. See Ken Anderson's book *How to Change Your Drinking* for a very detailed explanation of controlled drinking strategies.

Moderation

This option has a lot of wiggle room! What is moderate use for you may still seem excessive to someone else, but it is *your* baseline that's important. Moderation means limiting yourself to less frequent use or a lesser amount than your usual. Moderation almost always starts with counting and measuring. Once you are comfortable with really *knowing* how much you're using, you can begin to lower your consumption to a level that helps you feel better about yourself and reduces harm. If you're smoking marijuana from morning till bedtime, moderation for you might be smoking a bowl in the morning and after lunch, then before bedtime—but not all day. If you are drinking eight beers at night, lowering that to five (if you are a man) or three (if you are a woman) would be a moderation plan. There are clear guidelines about what constitutes low-risk or moderate drinking (see the pamphlet "Rethinking Drinking" and book *Responsible Drinking,* or go to *www.moderation.org*), but those limits may be too strict for you. The next chapter of this book is the harm reduction substance use management guide for other drugs. (See also *www.erowid.org* and other listings in the Resources at the back of this book.)

Abstinence

Although just the sound of this word may make you sweat, you might decide that it would be best if you quit using *everything.* Then you don't have to pay attention to making sure that, if you quit drinking, you don't start smoking more pot. It also protects you from other kinds of drug substitutions that haven't worked for you in the past. Like quitting speed and finding that you are drinking eight cups of coffee a day. Or quitting heroin but drinking a lot or using benzos. But abstinence can also mean that you decide to quit only one or two of the drugs you use and continue with the others. This is often more difficult, because our tendency is to want to replace what we are now missing. If you decide to quit just one of your drugs, it will be important for you to make a *plan* about the remaining drugs rather than just let nature take its course.

All of this—decisions, plans, and change—takes an enormous amount of effort. We understand and respect that. This might be a good time to take a break. When you come back, the rest of the chapter will guide you through a self-evaluation and goal-setting process.

The Work of Change

Your Wish List

Change starts with a wish. It's not complicated. It doesn't have to be detailed. You can change your mind later. At this moment, how do you *wish* you would use each of your drugs? What is your vision of the ideal relationship with each of your drugs? What would you like to use more safely? What would you like to control better? What would you like to moderate? How about quitting—is there anything you would like to let go of? And last but

> Change starts with a wish.

not least, what would you like to leave just as it is for now?

The simple form on page 126 allows you to create your wish list of change. Use it to list each drug that you use, then list the concern or concerns related to each drug that you identified in Chapter 5. Finally, put an X in the box that represents what you would like to do about your drug now or in the near future. You can give yourself more space to fill out the form by downloading and printing it out (see the end of the Contents for information on printing additional copies).

If you would prefer, you may use the continuum steps to set your goals (see page 127). Use the blank space inside each step to lay out details of how you might use more safely, control your use, moderate, or abstain. (You will get more information about how to accomplish these goals in the next chapter, but you might already have some good ideas.)

You have now established your *goals*. You know what you want to achieve for each of the drugs that concern you. You can always change your mind later, but we will carry on in the next section with an assessment of how *ready* you are to start working toward these goals.

Your Readiness to Change:
What Are You Saying to Yourself?

In Chapter 6 we introduced you to the language of change. What you are saying to yourself or others about each of your drugs is a good indication of your readiness to do something about your drug use. In this section we ask

My Change Wish List

Drug	Your concerns	Goal			
		Safety	Control	Moderation	Abstinence	Nothing

My Harm Reduction Continuum

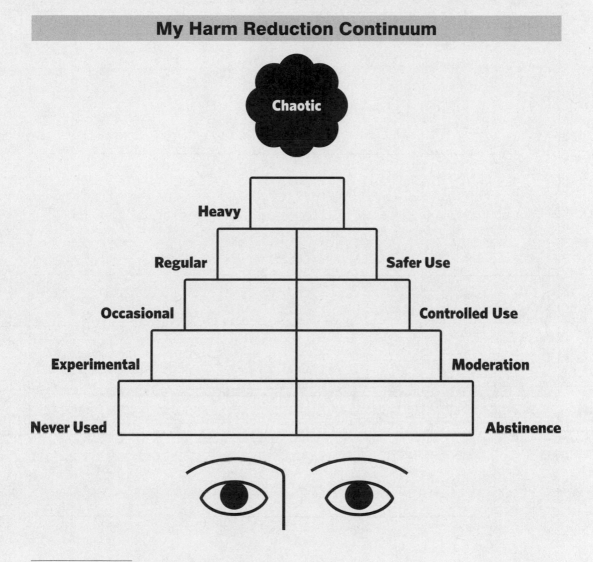

you to write down the language you are using about each drug. It is crucial that you listen to yourself with kindness, value your own thoughts and feelings, and trust yourself to make the decisions that are right for you. On the next page is a chart to help you write down your thoughts and words. Consider the drug issues that you listed in "My Change Wish List." List them here. Then reflect on what words come to mind when you think or talk about these issues.

What I Am Saying to Myself

Drug Problem	The Words I Am Saying to Myself: Change or Sustain?

The thoughts and words you wrote down will tell you where you are on the Readiness Ruler shown below. Put each issue where it belongs—in the low readiness, the moderate readiness, or the high readiness box. It doesn't matter what is on your list—your substance use, things that surround your use, or other issues that are causing you harm and need attention before you can even think about changing your relationship with drugs.

Importance, Readiness, and Confidence

On the next page is another Readiness Ruler, one that will drill deeper into all the factors that indicate readiness to do something. It invites you to put importance and readiness together with the level of *confidence* that you have about succeeding in your change efforts.

> The *importance* of an issue and your *confidence* in how effectively you can do something about it will help you assess your overall readiness more accurately.

My Readiness Ruler

Are you not prepared to change, already changing, or somewhere in the middle?

0 1 2	3 4 5 6	7 8 9 10

☐ **I don't know**

Not prepared   **Already changing**

My Complex Readiness Ruler

I would like to make changes to : _

_ _

IMPORTANCE

On a scale of 0 to 10, with 0 meaning "not important at all," and 10 meaning "couldn't be more important," here's how important making these changes are to me:

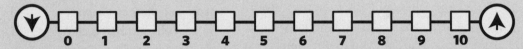

READINESS

On a scale of 0 to 10, with 0 meaning "not ready at all," and 10 meaning "couldn't be more ready," here's how ready I am to start making these changes:

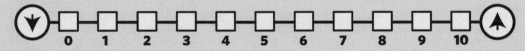

CONFIDENCE

On a scale of 0 to 10, with 0 meaning "not confident at all," and 10 meaning "couldn't be more confident," here's how confident I am that I can make these changes:

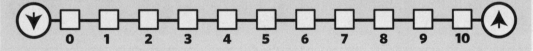

For example, if you have failed a drug test for your school sports team, it is important to you to quit smoking pot. You can't get away with timing your use to beat the drug test because pot stays in your system for a long time. Because your team is important to you, you feel motivated—you feel ready. But you have smoked pot since you were 15. You have no idea *how* to go about quitting. That means your confidence in your ability—your self-efficacy—is low. So despite how ready you feel, you aren't actually as ready as you would like to be.

The Stages of Change: Figuring Out What to Do

It's all very well to know how *ready* you are to work on your problem drugs and issues. But that doesn't tell you what to *do*. Identifying the stage of change for each issue will help. Because each stage of change is defined by your state of mind, it requires that you do different things. The table on the next page shows what we mean.

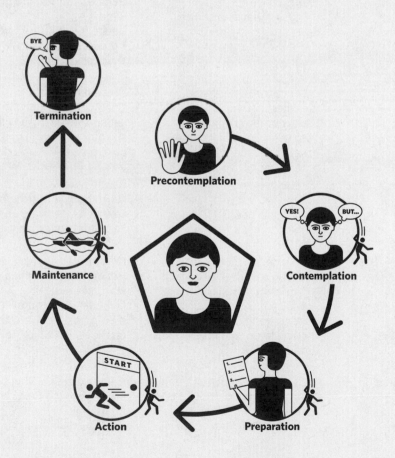

Stages of Change

Stage	State of Mind	What You Could Do
Precontemplation	Innocent, ignorant, resistant: "Who, me?" "I don't know what you mean." "I'm not interested in thinking about that."	• Talk to someone nonthreatening who you trust • Learn more about the drug/s you are using • Pay attention to your patterns
Contemplation	Ambivalent: "Yes, but." "On the one hand . . . on the other hand."	• Weigh the pros and cons • Focus on the reasons for change • Imagine letting go of something that you have relied on
Preparation	Decisive, determined, resigned: "I am going to . . . " "I will." "Oh, all right, I guess I have no choice."	• Get information about options • Decide what you are going to do • Define the steps required • Try out new behaviors • Make plans A and B
Action	Energized, determined, excited, nervous: "I am." "I can't believe I'm going to do this." "What if it doesn't work?"	• Do plan A • Change or work on the set and setting issues that surround the issue you have changed.
Relapse/recycling	Disappointed, frustrated: "Oh, no." "I blew it." "I'm in trouble now." "I'm never going to get it."	• Blame plan A • Learn from your experience • Switch to plan B • Take it off your wish list
Maintenance	Confident, proud, sad, feeling a void: "I've done it!" "I'm really proud of myself." "I miss _____." "It feels strange. What am I going to do with myself now?"	• Find new pleasures • Renew old friendships or start new ones • Deal with issues that emerge as you live with the changes you've made
Termination	Over it: "I'm done." "I haven't thought about _____ in years now." "Wow."	• Enjoy the rest of your life • Move on to the next challenge

There is no limit on how long you stay at each stage—no statute of limitations. All of us, if we thought about it, could name at least 10 things that we have contemplated for years and never managed to *do*—losing weight, telling our husband what we love about him even though he gets on our nerves, learning Spanish, calling our mother regularly. And we might contemplate them forever. The stages of change are not linear—you can revisit them many times. You can also change your mind. If so, go back and redo your wish list. As long as you are studious in your use of these tools, you are not ignoring your issues.

> There is no limit on how long you stay at each stage— no statute of limitations.

Your Stages of Change

Using the worksheet on page 135 (or see the end of the Contents for information on printing out additional copies), you can put each one of the drugs and issues from your wish list into the stage where you think it belongs. Use your change language and your Readiness Ruler as guides. In the third column, write down what you want to change—the goal you set on your wish list. First, look at Cheryl's example below.

Cheryl's Stages of Change		
Stage	**Drug/s or Issue/s**	**Goal and Steps**
Precontemplation		
Contemplation	Pills	<u>Abstinence</u> Pros and cons list Imagine what I will lose—how hard will it be? Focus a lot on positives of quitting Remember that I can change my mind
Preparation	Alcohol	<u>Moderation</u> Research moderation: Join an online chat at www.moderation.org or HAMS Plan A: follow the guidelines in the book <u>How to Change Your Drinking</u>

(continued)

Cheryl's Stages of Change *(continued)*		
Stage	**Drug/s or Issue/s**	**Goal and Steps**
Preparation	Alcohol	Try out different suggestions, one week at a time—don't extend the time yet
		Pick a strategy and make a plan
		Plan B: Sign up for CheckUp and Choices; do the CheckUp
		Set a date
Action		
Relapse/recycling		
Maintenance		
Termination		

Now, if you are ready, fill in the My Stages of Change worksheet for yourself. If you want, you can put the words that you are saying to yourself in the stage boxes.

If you are not a fan of boxes and lines, you might prefer to use the wheel on page 136 (and also available online—see the end of the Contents for information on printing out additional copies) to lay out your issues, goals, and steps.

You have just developed your change plan. We mentioned doing a pros and cons list as one of Cheryl's steps to resolve her ambivalence about quitting pills.

Working through Ambivalence: Weighing the Pros and Cons

The decisional balance, developed by two research psychologists in the 1970s to facilitate decision making, is a structure that can help you weigh "On the one hand . . . " and "on the other hand . . . " against each other. Comparing the pros and cons, finding the balance between the advantages and the disadvantages of change, and of continuing on as usual, gets at all the reasons to change *and the reasons not to*. You can see how this works in Cheryl's case. We do a pros and cons analysis of her pills because, although she has a wish to quit (it's really a "should"), her state of mind is ambivalent.

My Stages of Change

Stage	Drug/s or Issue/s	Goal and Steps
Precontemplation		
Contemplation		
Preparation		
Action		
Relapse/recycling		
Maintenance		
Termination		

My Stages of Change Wheel

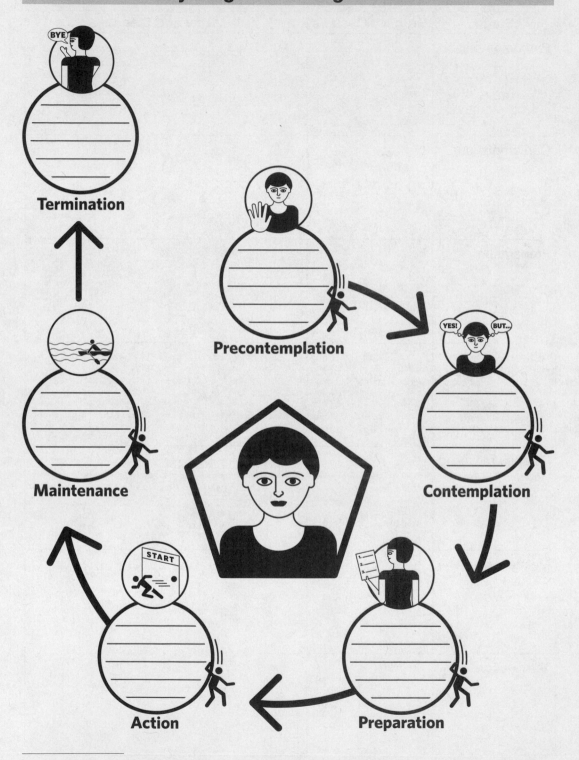

Cheryl's Pros and Cons		
Options	**Pros**	**Cons**
Quit using pills	Avoid getting caught (and risking my license).	It will be really hard.
	I will have to manage job stress in a more constructive way.	I might start drinking even more.
	I will have to face my relationship issues head on.	Nothing else has ever made my anxiety go away—I can't imagine finding anything else that will work as well.
Keep using pills	Helps me reduce my alcohol intake.	I could overdose.
	I'm more mellow, less argumentative.	I am going to find it harder and harder to get them.
	No hangovers.	I could get caught and lose my license.

While the pros of quitting and the cons of continuing (as well as the cons of quitting and the pros of continuing) might seem to be mirror images of each other, they are not. The pros and cons of each are considered from a different perspective and call up different thoughts and feelings. While there is some overlap, there are distinctions, which adds to the complexity of Cheryl's dilemma. This is good. Dilemmas are dilemmas *because* they are complicated.

Your Decisional Balance

Use the simple form on the next page (also available online—see the end of the Contents for information on printing out additional copies). Pick any issue on your list for which you are in contemplation. Once you've put together your lists of benefits and costs, you can compare them. On one hand, you have the *pros* of changing. On the other hand, you have the *cons* of changing. Then you have another list—the *pros* of not changing and the *cons* of not changing. Your goal in the decisional balance is to bring both sides into focus.

The easy part is creating the list. The hard part is figuring out how much each item *weighs* to determine which side "wins." This could take months or years of pondering. Following the laws of both physics and human experience, the **benefits** of changing will eventually have to outweigh the **costs** before you're persuaded to do anything.

Decisional Balance Worksheet

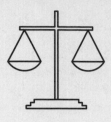

NOT TO CHANGE	TO CHANGE
Things I like about _____	**Things I don't like about** _____
Difficult things about changing my use	**Good things about changing my use**

What's Next?

Are you ready to make a more specific plan? Things that you are ready to change now require a plan. Most of us don't just "do it." We also need to experiment with different options to figure out what fits us best and is likely to be sustainable. In the next chapter we will give you information about substance use management, which is at the core of harm reduction practice. The chapter is full of very specific recommendations about what you do to manage each drug—how to reduce harm, control, moderate, and quit. As we suggested in this chapter, when you are preparing for change, develop plans by trying a few things out and seeing if you like them. The next chapter will give you many ideas to consider and practice.

Not quite ready? As we've said before, if things start seeming too hard or overwhelming, just put the book down and grab a bite to eat or watch TV. You can come back to it later.

You don't have to quit to change.

Trust yourself to make the decisions that are right for you.

You get to change your mind.

8 Substance Use Management

*Substance Use Management spans the
divide between chaotic, out of control
drug use and a drug-free life.*
—Dan Bigg, founder and director
of the Chicago Recovery Alliance

Wanting to change, being motivated to change, and hoping that you'll change aren't exactly road maps. In the spirit of Just Say Know, this chapter is about *how* to change.

If you have not yet decided to be abstinent, have decided to quit but you're just not ready, or if you've decided to keep using but want to manage your drug use better, the resources available to you are pretty slim. While there are many guides to alcohol moderation (see the Resources), you have to piece it together for other drugs—from your using community, websites, health alerts, and your own ups and downs. The purpose of this chapter is to fill that gap (actually, that's the point of this whole book!). *Substance use management* (SUM) is your guide to controlled use and moderation for all drugs. This information can help you manage your drug use. It might also save your life. *But it is not a guarantee.*

The wisdom guiding substance use management is ancient. As described in Chapter 2, rituals and controls typically surrounded the use of strong substances. The Renaissance physician Paracelsus pointed out, "The poison is in the dose," which is just as true for botulin (now used to reduce facial wrinkles) as it is for nicotine, alcohol, or ketamine. When physicians, philosophers, and the general public expressed concern about drug use, it had to do with the amount used, the "dose." Eventually, how much a person used *over time* became just as important as how much he or she consumed at any *one* time.

This is the attitude of those who practice substance use management. It's not *what* you use necessarily, but how, when, where, and how much you use that contributes to either harm or safety. This is the wisdom that eventually emerged out of research as the Drug, Set, Setting model. You used it in Chapter 5 to identify the concerns you have about the various aspects of your relationship with drugs. It is equally useful to guide your substance use change plan.

Substance use management relies on your ability and willingness to *observe* yourself. It also assumes that you, and only you, are responsible for what you put into your body. It is designed to empower you to take charge of your use. SUM is based on three principles:

1. Being *honest* with yourself about your drug use and the impact of drugs in your life.

2. Being *willing* to study your drugs and learn new skills.

3. Implementing those *skills* to help you make concrete, beneficial changes in your alcohol or other drug use.*

This chapter offers a structure to guide you in how to use more wisely and more safely. We give you general guidelines about how SUM works. Many of the suggestions offered here are derived from books about drugs, from websites, public health pamphlets, harm reduction videos, and professional books and lectures, and from our clients and our experience as therapists. It is general information that is publicly available. It is unlikely to cover all that might be involved in your particular drug use patterns. That would take half a library, but we'll give you several other resources to check out. In conjunction with the information on each class of drugs at the end of the book and the other sources we recommend, you can develop a solid substance use management plan.

Substance Use Management Using Drug, Set, Setting

Drug, Set, Setting offers a great structure to guide your efforts to control, in some way, your substance use. Norman Zinberg managed to capture all of the elements that lead to each person's unique relationship with drugs— detailed understanding of each drug, the person's motivations, and the extent to which the setting encourages control or lack of control. The drug, set, and setting elements of your drug use, the concerns that you highlighted, and your substance use goals are the starting point for your work in this chapter.

---

*You can order harm reduction and safer injection information and a video on safer injection techniques from the Chicago Recovery Alliance and pamphlets from the Harm Reduction Coalition in New York.

A Disclaimer

We are not medical doctors and therefore are not qualified to give medical advice or prescriptions. If you have a harm-reduction-friendly doctor who will advise you about the interaction of "street" drugs with prescribed medication, seek out him or her. If you don't have access to professional advice, you'll have to put together a plan for yourself. Look for other drug users to talk to, but *only those you think do a good job of taking care of themselves and who seem to be educated about the drugs they use*. There are many people in the harm reduction movement you can talk to—the Harm Reduction Coalition in New York or Oakland is a great resource. A needle exchange program is a good place to go, too, even if you aren't an injection drug user. People there know a lot about most drugs. There are, of course, many websites that offer accurate information about drugs. We'll list some of those in the Resources.

    We are also not attorneys and cannot protect you from legal sanctions! Most of the drugs we are talking about are illegal. Each state has different laws regarding possession, sale, and so forth. We suggest you do some research on your own, look at the Drug Policy Alliance website, and become familiar with the legal harms that you could suffer from using.

While most of the details of managing your substance use fall under how you manage the drugs themselves, managing your set and setting makes it easier to manage your drugs. Set and setting have a bigger impact on your drug use than the drugs themselves do. We will start, therefore, with how you handle those aspects of your drug use, then move into the details of managing your drugs. Bring with you the concerns you identified in Chapter 5, concerns about yourself, your mind-set, and the settings. And bring your safety, control, moderation, and abstinence goals for each of your drugs.

Set

Most of our focus on *you*—your mind-set about drugs and when you use drugs—comes in the next chapter about how to take care of yourself. Here we want to introduce you to some ideas about to how to manage yourself. Your motivation for using, your expectations of what will happen when you use, your personality, and your health have a large impact on the quality of each drug experience. Taking control of your*self* is the first step toward controlling your drug use.

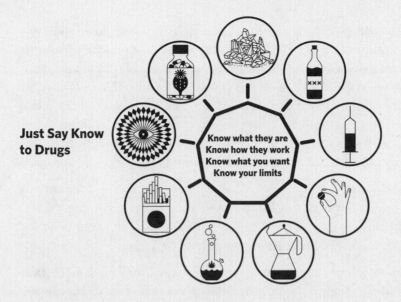

Just Say Know to Drugs

Know what they are
Know how they work
Know what you want
Know your limits

Just Say Know

What Do You Want?

To party, have fun, improve your concentration, feel closer to others, see the world differently, sleep, numb out, get wasted? Knowing what you want to get out of each experience of using is one of the best ways of taking control. For each of your drugs, think about what you hope to feel: a little buzzed or relaxed, really high, or totally out of it? Another way of saying this is: Are you using for recreation, for intoxication, or for oblivion? This is your motivation for using. If you find the right drug, you expect it to achieve what you want. But what if you want to get just a little buzzed, but then you eat too many bites of cannabis brownie and get wasted? Your motivation and expectation didn't match up. That's why knowing what you're taking and how strong it is becomes important. Also, your motivation may change at times. Maybe you just want a little buzz during the week but want to get totally out of it on Saturday night. So you pay a lot more attention to the type of drug, the amount, and the potency during the week, and less attention on the weekends.

Pay Attention to What You Are Doing Now

When your use is habitual, you might stop paying attention to whether it's actually doing what you want (bringing pleasure, numbing pain, and so forth). There might be a lot of other things that you're *not* doing, too—things that you actually *want* to do!

- *Measure and count*: Measuring means measuring your dose; counting refers to the number of doses. Whether it's the number of standard drinks or your own definition of a "dose" (hits on a bong, E, lines of coke), it's important to know what your usual pattern is if you want to be able to change it. Since it's difficult to know if the three lines of coke you snorted last week are the same "dose" as the three lines you snorted this week, counting is an inexact science. As we've said before, if you have a large enough supply on hand to last you through several uses, then counting becomes more accurate.

- *Pay attention to how you feel before you use*: Feeling great and wanting to celebrate is different from feeling lousy and wanting to get rid of that feeling. If you pay attention to how you feel before you start, you can begin to notice what state of mind lends itself to better control.

- *Reevaluate whether you got what you wanted*: We know it's hard to take a close look at your high once it's over. Sometimes you want to bask in the glow. Other times you want to forget all about it. Or you're moving on to the next one already. But you'll get more out of the next time if you can assess how things went the last time.

> Know what you want and what it will take to achieve it.

What Kind of Person Are You?

A risk taker? Impulsive? Carefree? Timid and cautious? Rebellious? A joiner who is inclined to try what everyone around you is doing? Someone who prefers to be alone? If your style of using fits your personality, you will have to study your relationship with drugs closely. If you like going out on the edge, and yet you want to cut way back, you will have to figure out other ways to get there. If drugs help you go inside yourself, if they protect you, how else can you feel enclosed and protected? This is where revisiting your record of the harms and benefits (see Chapters 2 and 3), as well as your decisional balance (see Chapter 7), will help you use your rational self to argue with your emotional self and come to some compromise.

Take Care of Yourself

The Basics

Eat, sleep, breathe, stay warm, find love.

Your Health

Get treatment for physical and mental health issues. That can be hard because of policies in many places against prescribing medications to drug users. Do your best. Ask for referrals.

The Things That Drive Your Use

Anxiety in social situations. Traumatic memories that flood you. Desire for belonging that clouds your judgment. These are specific issues that you can work on so they don't drive your use. Self-help books, talking to friends, or therapy can help you reduce the "drive" to use.

Putting It All Together: Managing Triggers and Cravings

This is what it really comes down to. In any given moment, you might be faced with a decision about whether to pick up a drink or a drug or not. Triggers are all of the cues that remind you of your drugs. Craving is the feeling and the sensation that you sometimes get in response to those cues.

> Remember, just because you *think* about speed, heroin, alcohol, or a cigarette doesn't mean that you will automatically *want* it.

Sights, smells, people, places, and events *stimulate* us. We have what amounts to a chemical reaction, no different from salivating when we see a steaming plate of our favorite pasta or a chocolate cake. It is a physical reaction that comes with the thought "Mmmmm, that looks *so* good" followed by a feeling of desire. If you are an impulsive person, you will find it difficult to resist a craving. You will probably need to put things in place in your setting to keep yourself from calling your dealer or running out to the corner store.

A long day at work or a fight with a friend might bring on feelings we want to get rid of. Being with friends at a concert, especially with the smell of weed in the air, might trigger a desire to smoke. Finishing a project at work is cause for celebration. We're kind of like machines in this regard: something triggers our memories of using or causes an intense feeling; we then have a wish to do something about these feelings—this is the craving. Then we either give in to it or not.

There are many great techniques for managing cravings. Most involve either distraction, substitution, or location change. One that we like is timing the impulse. When you first feel the wish to use, check the time and write it down if you can. Then just stand still. Don't do anything. Or if it's easier, move around, adjust the window shades, get a drink of water. Distract yourself for a while. *The impulse will go away.* As soon as you notice that you forgot about using, check the time. Was it 1 minute or 10? This is your time frame for controlling yourself. You can say to yourself, "If I can wait 10 minutes, this urge to use will go away." If the urge comes back, do it again. You're trying to teach yourself, *"This urge will go away whether or not I use!"*

> "This urge will go away whether or not I use!"

Some people refer to this as "urge surfing"—riding out the wave of craving until you reach the shore again. You can use our method of focusing, other mindfulness practices, meditation, strenuous exercise, chores, or any number of other disciplines and distractions.

Setting

Where you use and with whom can either increase or decrease the riskiness of using any particular drug. As we mentioned before, shooting drugs under the freeway or in a public bathroom makes it harder to take your time and use good hygiene. Consider these aspects of the setting in which you use.

Where Do You Use?

Safe Surroundings

Does where you use facilitate a good experience or contribute to a negative one? Do you have a place to clean any equipment and keep it sterile? If you use outside, are you safe from the police so you don't have to rush your hit? Is your home depressing, making you want to get higher? Can you *see* what you're taking? Swallowing a bunch of pills that you can't even see and drinking out of a bottle that you haven't been in control of are sure ways to let the

> Try to use where and when you can have some privacy, light, and access to water.

setting control you rather than the other way around.

Setting is just as important with alcohol as it is with drugs. You might drink at home and be fine, but if you drink when you're out, you have a tendency to get into fights. Or you find that if you drink with friends, it's a pleasant experience and you don't drink as much. When you're home alone, you tend to get weepy and drink too much. Get to know yourself in different situations. You'll find it easier to manage your drug or alcohol use if you're in charge of *where* you use.

> Getting to know yourself in different situations will help you stay in charge of where you use and more easily manage your use.

With Whom Do You Use?

Your Using Culture

If you are a user of illegal drugs, it's important to know how educated and thoughtful the people you use with are about safety, dosage, and optimal experience. Often people haven't been well informed about methods of control and moderation, which could make the difference between safety and harm and between positive and negative experiences.

The Customs in Your Using Environment

A lot of drug and alcohol use is social. Therefore your environment might need some changes for substance use management to really work for you—not only the places and the situations in which you use but also the people with whom you use can be triggers to use or produce cravings. If you want to reduce the amount you're using, see how difficult this might be to manage in your particular environment. If your friends are big consumers, it could be anything from awkward to virtually impossible to control how much you use. Try avoiding these people until you've reduced your use. That way, you will have some success under your belt and you can transfer your learning to your old situation.

Are You Triggered by Being Alone or with Certain People?

- If you're a heavy user when alone and moderate in public, consider restricting yourself to social situations to reduce the amount you use.

- If you use more heavily in situations that make you feel bad—Sunday dinners with your quarreling family, for example—avoid them for a while if possible.

- Beware, however, if you are a heroin user. If you switch settings or supply, use a smaller dose at first and, if you can, have someone with you to watch your back and call 911 if needed. Again, having naloxone

> More overdoses occur when regular users use in unfamiliar environments or alone.

with you can save your life if there is another person there to administer it.

Drug

Most of the techniques of SUM fall under the drug umbrella—changing the route of administration, the amount and/or the frequency, and the combinations you use. We organize all of the following according to the goals you set for each of your drugs (safety, controlled use/moderation, and abstinence). Bring that list (My Harm Reduction Continuum), as well as your specific change goals and steps from the last chapter, with you into this section.

Safety

The most dangerous risks of substance misuse are fatal overdose, accidents, and violence. Other serious risks include health problems such as stroke and heart attacks, disease transmission, infections, and dangerous withdrawal symptoms. While perhaps not immediately fatal, these dangers could land you in the hospital in the short term and cause difficult health conditions down the road.

Overdose

To overdose simply means that you have taken too much—you have gone over the dose that your body can handle. Sedating drugs like opioids, pills, and alcohol slow respiration to dangerous levels. Stimulating drugs can cause strokes, heart attacks, and hyperthermia.

Opioid Overdose

When you overdose, you "fall out," meaning you become unconscious, can't be shaken awake, and your breathing is shallow. Lack of response to a sternal rub (rubbing your knuckles over the chest bone) means a person has overdosed and it is time to act!

1. Start rescue breathing immediately (this is the breathing part of CPR).
2. Administer naloxone. Naloxone (Narcan) quickly reverses what could be a fatal experience. It actually interrupts a high by kicking

Overdose

You are at greatest risk of overdose if you:

- Mix drugs (even opioids and stimulants used together increase OD risk).

- Don't pay attention to the drugs you're using, know their speed of onset, peak impact, effect with other drugs, and length of action.

- Use alone.

- Shoot drugs but don't do your own shot or test your shot, especially with a new supply.

- Forget that alcohol poisoning can be fatal and just try to sleep it off.

- Take drugs you don't know about.

your opioids off the opioid receptors in your brain and blocking any further absorption of whatever drug you took. (You will be in withdrawal when you come to.) The dramatic increase in opioid overdose in this country has made naloxone more widely available for home use, instead of just by medical professionals, so that friends can take care of friends. Naloxone is distributed by hundreds of programs throughout the world to people using drugs. Some emergency medical technicians and police also carry it, as do hospital emergency rooms. Many states have passed laws allowing anyone to purchase naloxone at a pharmacy. It comes in both injectable and intranasal forms. Get some for yourself and learn how to use it. Teach friends and family members. **Be aware that naloxone can wear off** before your opioid dose, so make sure you remain under observation and that another naloxone dose is administered if you start to become unconscious again.

3. Call 911. Readminister Narcan if necessary.

4. To *prevent* overdose, test your shot before you take it all so you can make sure of its potency. Do your best to know if your pills are really what they say they are.

Alcohol Poisoning

Alcohol poisoning occurs when you drink too much too fast, eventually slowing your respiration to the point of potential death. If someone passes out, don't leave the person to sleep it off.

Don't Be Afraid to Call 911 or Take Your Friends to a Hospital!

Getting in trouble is better than dying. Many states have Good Samaritan laws that will protect you. But if you're going to get the law involved, dump your illegal drugs before calling and minimize the harm to yourself. If you don't want to stay around because you've had legal problems before, call 911, perform rescue breathing, wait to hear the siren, then put your friend on his or her side and go. Or, better: When you call 911, simply tell them the truth: "My friend is having trouble breathing." That will cue emergency personnel to come quick.

1. Try to rouse the person using a sternal rub.

2. Make sure he is lying on his side so he does not inhale his vomit.

3. Call 911 if you cannot rouse him.

Stroke, Heart Attack, Hyperthermia

In general, stimulants increase the risk of stroke and heart attack, while drugs like ecstasy lead to hyperthermia because of the increase in activity levels (like dancing) in hot places, often with alcohol and without enough water. Most problems are caused by taking too much of a drug too quickly, taking dose after dose without waiting for the drug to get pro-

> The problem is, the *sensation* of being high passes before the *drug* does.

cessed and excreted. The problem is, the *sensation* of being high passes before the *drug* does. This is how it happens when you are partying. You're chasing a high, not paying attention to your body.

Cannabis Alert

Research indicates that some people—primarily men between the ages of 40 and 50—have an increased risk of heart attack within 30 minutes after using. Cannabis temporarily increases heart rate and can be dangerous if you have an underlying and/or unknown heart problem.

Disease Transmission, Infection, and Safe Injection

Injection drug use puts you at risk for blood-borne disease transmission—HIV and hepatitis if you are sharing equipment. It is also a possible source of infection because you are puncturing the skin, which allows whatever germs there are in the environment or on your skin to get into your bloodstream. Infections can cause abscesses and can also get to your heart. Here are several harm reduction techniques:

1. Use a clean needle for each shot. Not only the needle, but the cooker and cotton, tie, and your skin at the injection site (keep alcohol wipes) should be absolutely clean. It's risky to share any of your equipment with others. If you don't have a choice, remember that sharing needles requires careful hygiene with bleach and water to be safe.

2. Rotate injection sites to let puncture wounds heal.

3. Learn how to shoot accurately in different locations. See *www.harm reduction.org/drugs-and-drug-users/drug-tools/getting-off-right* and the Chicago Recovery Alliance website at *www.anypositivechange.org/bvcsi.html* for guidelines on safe injection.

4. A *new* needle for each shot is ideal but sometimes hard to manage. Each use of the needle makes it duller and causes more damage to your veins. A rule of thumb: **If it hurts, pull out the needle.** An IV injection should not cause pain (the drug might burn, but the needle itself shouldn't hurt). If it does, you've missed the vein and may be in a nerve, an artery, or just sensitive tissue. Injection wounds are best treated like any other injury that swells—ice for the first 24 hours, then apply heat to heal. See the abscess identification guide at *www.anypositivechange.org*.

5. If you're using a drug of unknown potency, test a little before you give yourself the whole shot. It'll act as an early warning signal if it's too strong or mixed with toxic junk.

Shoot safe.

The bottom line: Shoot safe. Or switch to safer routes of administration—snorting, smoking, or swallowing. Sure, you won't get quite the same bang for your "buck," but you might last longer.

Withdrawal

If you are physiologically dependent (you get sick or shaky when you try to quit), going "cold turkey" or "kicking" could be dangerous. Sudden withdrawal from alcohol, benzodiazepines (such as Valium, Xanax, Ativan, Klonopin), or barbiturates can cause seizures, DTs, or death. If this is the case, you would be better off with medical detoxification until your tolerance is lowered safely, especially if you have HIV, diabetes, a heart condition, or other problems that are made worse by stress. If you try to "tough it out," your chances of succeeding go down and your risk of medical problems goes up. The point is to lower the amount enough to make a difference without causing a medical crisis.

Miserable as it is (severe flu-like symptoms for many people), detox from opioids is not dangerous, but it can be ineffective because of the fierce craving to stop dope sickness. Medication detox using methadone or buprenorphine is one option. A lot has been written about the use of acupuncture for both detoxification and managing cravings. Dr. Michael Smith of the Lincoln Hospital Acupuncture Program in the Bronx was one of the people who developed "AcuDetox," an acupuncture method that consists

> Acupuncture and other nurturing activities can help you manage detox and withdrawal and manage cravings.

of placing five needles in points in your ear. You might also try massage, yoga, and other types of nurturing activities to help manage your withdrawal.

Controlled Use and Moderation

Safety is vitally important as a foundation of harm reduction, but people's goals usually involve achieving a level of use that can *fit into* their life, not disrupt it.

Control simply means being intentional about what you are using, when, and where, then having a plan, making rules, and following through. Much of this work is done by focusing on yourself (set) and taking charge of the situation (setting). Control is not about an overall amount—you can use quite heavily and risk significant consequences, although usually people are intending to be safe and stay out of trouble. It is about your intention and behavior. Some people drink nightly, two glasses of wine with dinner or a cocktail after work followed by a brandy after dinner. Others plan a monthly binge where they go out with friends and get wasted. They don't drive and don't have any responsibilities the next day. Same with speed, recreational (as opposed to maintenance) heroin use, cocaine, cannabis, and anything else. Exactly the same rules apply.

Moderation, on the other hand, refers to *low-risk* drug use and comes with an actual recommended amount of a drug. This is easy with legal drugs— they are well researched and their risks well known. Alcohol moderation for men is considered to be no more than 14 standard drinks per week, on no more than four occasions, with no more than four drinks consumed on any occasion. For women, it is three standard drinks no more than three times a week, limited to three drinks per occasion. (Government health recommendations are slightly lower.) For cigarettes, of course, it is as little as possible, with none being the recommended amount. Caffeine is usually limited by the level of stimulation you can take before you get shaky. In the case of illegal drugs, you have to work it out based on an assessment of physical risk and impact on your life. Moderation means *low risk,* and that depends on your health and on your circumstances. If you have hepatitis, 14 or 9 drinks a week is probably too much. If you are a pilot or a health care professional, moderate means *no* drinking within 12 hours of a work shift. You have to adapt your moderation plan to fit your circumstances.

To create a control or moderation plan, think of each drug separately, but also about the combinations you use and how they mask or intensify one another's effects. Your plan for controlling or moderating your use can include changing the route of administration, the amount, and the frequency; you can also consider medication-assisted control.

Changing the Route of Administration (How You Take the Drug)

Any way you use can be made more or less safe. You can swallow a drug, smoke it, snort it, put it in other mucous membranes (eyes, nose, butt), inhale the fumes, rub it on your skin, or use a needle to put it in a vein, a muscle, or under your skin. Some drugs are "naturally" taken only in certain forms. Alcohol is swallowed. Nitrous oxide is a gas, so it is inhaled. Other drugs cannot be taken in oral form because stomach acids eat them up. Most drugs, however, can be prepared in several different ways and used by various routes of administration. Since control and moderation involve becoming more conscious and intentional, switching from one way of using a drug to another can be useful just to heighten your awareness of what you are doing.

If you smoke, be aware that for short-acting drugs like cocaine (and, of course, nicotine), smoking is the fastest way for the drug to get to your brain, but the high doesn't last long. That will make you want to do more and more, faster and faster. (This is when overdose becomes a risk.) You might want to switch to a slower route of administration.

If you inject, you will get the largest percentage of the dose to your brain and pretty quickly. It is a very efficient method, but because of the risks associated with IV drug use, you might consider switching. Follow the safe injection guidelines on page 151. To control or moderate, you might consider switching to a safer route of administration because it will eliminate the risks of injection. If you decide to smoke, see the caution above.

If you snort, take care of your poor nose. Heroin is not particularly abrasive, but cocaine and speed are. Mix the powder with a little water and spray it in. Or rub the inside of your nose with vitamin E oil before using. Crushed pills won't pass into the blood vessels in your nose very well, so you might as well just swallow them or mix them in water and drink.

If you drink or eat, you are taking drugs in the slowest and least efficient method. But some drugs are best ingested orally. Drinking alcohol on a full stomach will extend the time it takes for the alcohol to be absorbed, which will keep your judgment clearer for making decisions about the next drink. But if what you really want is a quick buzz, have the first drink on an empty stomach and start eating after you begin to feel the effects, to slow down the process for the next drinks. Food does not make such a difference with other drugs. But it is very good for your health and indicates that you are balancing your drug-using life with other normal human behaviors!

When eating other drugs, Just Say Know:

- *Cannabis*: Know the potency of the cannabis products you are eating, get recipes from friends, eat a little (a quarter of a brownie, for example) and wait an hour to see how you feel before eating a little more. If you don't have much time, switch to smoking.

- *Pills*: The important thing to know is whether they are standard legal drugs or have been manufactured in a home lab. You can look up standard drugs in textbooks and online to see what you've got and how strong they are. You can also research how a particular drug interacts with others. For homemade pills, such as ecstasy or LSD, you'll have to ask around. Does anyone know what it is and how strong it is? Has anyone taken this particular pill before? Take only one if you're not sure. You can always do more later.

Changing the Amount or the Frequency

Less is more. You are more likely to actually *enjoy* your drug experience if you don't do it all the time or in large quantities. We can't be comprehensive

> Some drugs, or drug use patterns, lend themselves to changing the amount—tapering—others to changing the frequency.

here, but the following guidelines should help structure your thinking. Use them in conjunction with the information in the section on drugs at the end of the book, but also keep in mind that websites and social media are the best way to stay up to date with drug information that can guide your decisions.

There is overlap, but here are some guidelines:

- *If you are physiologically dependent,* meaning that you have been drinking or using for a while, your body and brain have adapted to the drug's effects, and you have to use more to get the same high. You have developed *tolerance.* Quitting will be harder and might be dangerous. See the section on withdrawal on page 152. Reducing the frequency of your use will be hard too. If you are a daily and dependent opioid, alcohol, or pill user, you are not going to take days off. If you are a daily and habitual caffeine or tobacco user, this is also unlikely. You are going to be more successful, and more comfortable, reducing the amount, or the dose.

- *If you're not physiologically dependent,* the best and easiest way to decrease tolerance is to quit for a while. Even a few days can make a difference, but a few weeks is better. This time off will give you a chance to decide how much you will use once you start again. **Be aware that, if injecting opioids, starting up again after some period of abstinence is a major risk factor for overdose. Always test your dose before injecting the full amount.** If you don't quit, you can space out the time between doses. Short-acting drugs, and drugs that you use occasionally—stimulants, hallucinogens, ecstasy, dissociative anesthetics, and inhalants—lend themselves well to frequency reduction. Cannabis can go either way.

Starting on a Reduction Plan—Changing the Amount

Once you know how much you're drinking or using, you can begin a *reduction plan*:

1. Start by writing the details of your current use in a journal or notebook—how much, how often, and so forth. There are a number of mobile apps that you can use for alcohol. Keep track for a week or

two. That way you will know how much you typically use and can keep better track of your progress as you change.

2. The general rule of thumb is "Start low and slow until you know." This means cutting down a little at a time so as to reduce the stress on your body. Stay at each new level until it feels comfortable or normal to you.

3. Be patient. You might notice that as you cut down, you won't be able to do it as quickly later as you could at the beginning. It's like dieting—it's easier to lose the first 10 pounds than the last 5. You'll know if your efforts are working not only by how you feel, but also by checking back with your journal to see the difference in your use over time.

> The rule of thumb for reducing the amount of a drug you use is "Start low and slow until you know."

This is a good time to revisit your step-down plan in My Harm Reduction Continuum on page 127. In Chapter 7 you set goals for each drug. Now you can fill in more details about how you might achieve each goal. Here are some examples of how you can do this with different drugs:

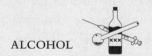

ALCOHOL

When you start drinking, have a pen and paper handy, use your phone or tablet, or write on your arm. Put a penny on the bar or in your pocket for each drink. Count the number of "drinks" in each of the drinks you consume (if you put two shots of vodka in orange juice, that's two drinks). If you typically have eight beers when you go out, try having only seven (or five). If you drink Manhattans, try what a friend in New York calls a "reverse Manhattan" (flip the ratio of whiskey to vermouth). Start with a large glass of water or juice before your first drink. Have some food. Then drink a glass of water after each alcoholic beverage. (Since a hangover is partly a result of dehydration, you will feel *way* better in the morning.) Drink slowly. If you really enjoy feeling the first drink, go ahead. You can do your controlling later. If you have a couple of drinks at lunch, then end up drinking for most of the rest of the day and evening, try delaying the first drink for an hour. Or stop drinking at lunch for a week or two. Now you're drinking only at night.

CANNABIS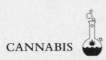

First, figure out the amount you are using. Know your product. In states where marijuana is legal, that is easy. Otherwise, know your dealer. Count your dose: one hit off a pipe or bong, half a joint, one-quarter of an edible, and so forth. Then decide whether you can live with a smaller dose and what that dose might be. If you don't live in a state that allows the sale and use of marijuana, test your dose to see how much you are getting. Because cannabis doesn't have a significant withdrawal syndrome unless you quit after heavy use, you can decrease the amount pretty easily.

STIMULANTS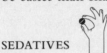

The percentage of active drug (say, speed) is likely to be different in each batch, so if you have a stash, you can cut back by first writing down how much how often, then decreasing that usual dose to a comfortable amount. If you use speed to party and play, however, changing the frequency of use will be easier than changing the amount.

SEDATIVES

Count the number of pills you take at any one time and reduce it by a small percentage so that you don't go into withdrawal—perhaps by one if you are using five a day. For pills bought on the street in larger quantities, you can test one and be fairly confident that the rest of the batch will be the same strength. As with other drugs to which you are tolerant, decide on a reduction schedule, then see how you feel. Benzos are a class of drug that has a potentially dangerous withdrawal syndrome. A little shaky is probably not dangerous, but if you start to sweat or feel nauseated and you're shaking quite a bit, or if you feel confused or panicky, you

> Benzos have a potentially dangerous withdrawal syndrome.

need medical assistance. **In fact, if you feel confused or are nauseated, you should go to an emergency room.** Then you'll have to rethink your decision to try this on your own.

OPIOIDS (HEROIN OR PILLS)

Slowly reducing heroin might mean starting off at your usual eight-bag day and then using only seven and a half bags tomorrow. If you're not too uncomfortable, try doing only seven the next day. Of course this procedure depends on consistent potency, which is not the norm. Again, buying in larger quantities along with other using friends might help you predict the strength, but keep in mind that you also run the risk of being charged with possession for sale if you get caught.

CAFFEINE AND TOBACCO

We group these together because they are legal and both can be quantified easily. The easiest way to reduce your caffeine intake is to fool yourself! Mix three-fourths caffeinated coffee or diet soda with one-quarter decaf for a week. Then try half and half, then . . . well, you get it. If you're a regular cigarette smoker, you can plan a tapering schedule. Keep a log of when you smoke each cigarette. Then decide which ones are most important to you. You can use a scale of 1 to 10, for example. You might smoke every hour, but when you rank their importance, you realize that the smokes at 10:00 and 11:00 A.M. aren't really that important, nor is the one at 3 P.M. These are the ones to cut out first. Keep a record and congratulate yourself for every small change.

Reduce by Changing the Frequency

If you've tried to cut down on the amount you use and haven't had consistently good results, changing how *often* you use might work better. The fact is, the less often you use, the less chance you will have to experience harm over the long run. If you are a daily user, you've probably developed tolerance and physical dependence; going without becomes difficult or impossible. To change the frequency, *just start with any positive change as you define it for yourself!*

STIMULANTS

Crack, powder cocaine, and speed are particularly difficult to control amount-wise. Once you start, they create a compulsion to keep on going till you run out of money or collapse. Reducing frequency is usually the best way to get some control. Whatever your pattern is, find something to interrupt it. Go to a movie or library; hang out with people who don't use. Even if it just delays the start of using, you'll probably end up using less that day.

Going without is not going to feel good. You'll feel run down, hungry, and depressed. Pick a day when you don't have to do anything, don't use, and just let yourself complain and be miserable. *You don't have to be brave about this.* Or try the opposite. Pick a day that'll keep you busy and sufficiently distracted. Being home alone with nothing to do can make it harder to stick with your plan. Here are a few other tips:

1. End your weekend parties by noon Sunday if you have a job to get to Monday morning.

2. Limit the money you take out with you and leave your bank card at home.

3. Cut down your using episodes by 25%, 50%, or 75%—from daily to every other day, weekly to every other week or once a month, or from monthly to quarterly. Enjoy every minute when you do get high.

ENTHEOGENS (ECSTASY, HALLUCINOGENS, KETAMINE FOR SOME PEOPLE, AND DESIGNER DRUGS)

We often say less is more, and in the case of these drugs, less is more, but less often is even better! Think of each trip as a vacation. Plan. Anticipate. Savor each experience—keep a journal of your memories and remind yourself that even if you wait a month, that same great experience is waiting for you.

DISSOCIATIVE ANESTHETICS, DESIGNER DRUGS, AND INHALANTS

Ketamine, PCP, DXM, Spice, nitrous, and the many "designer drugs" are wild cards in terms of how they affect you over time. The less you do these drugs, the better.

Inhalants such as glue and gasoline cause real brain *damage,* not just changes. And not just sometimes. We'd like to tell you not to use them at all, but they might be your only way to get out of your head. So use as infrequently as possible, since no one knows of any really safe way to use them. You can reduce the risk somewhat by only breathing what goes into the air and not the other contaminants. Instead of huffing a soaked rag, put the rag (soaked or sprayed) into a paper bag and let it settle before breathing the fumes—this can prevent more hazardous particles from getting into your lungs.

Many of these drugs provide users with wonderful experiences—of closeness to others, hallucinatory visions, lessening of self-consciousness, or insights into oneself or the world. If you don't want to give up those experiences, try treasuring them more and pursuing them less.

Medication–Assisted Control

Naltrexone is the oral, nonemergency version of naloxone (discussed in the safety section of this chapter). It also comes in a monthly injection form. It is used to reduce the craving for alcohol and to block opioid drugs (thus rendering them ineffective). In the United States, naltrexone is usually prescribed to be taken every day. But in Europe, the Sinclair Method (for alcohol), where you take a dose 1 hour before you might be drinking, has been shown to be more effective in helping people reduce the amount they drink. The disincentive approach in the case of opioids is not a harm reduction methodology. The idea that, if you block pleasure, you will cure drug misuse indicates a complete misunderstanding of the complexity of people's relationship with drugs. It also suggests punitive intentions.

Acamprosate is a medication that is used to stabilize chemical imbalances in the brain when people withdraw from alcohol. It can help to reduce craving.

Cannabis, because it is less harmful than most drugs, might be a consideration for people who are getting into trouble with other drugs but can't face life without something to alter their consciousness. We realize this kind of drug substitution is highly controversial because of the legal status of marijuana and because there can be negative effects related to age, dosage, and setting. But if you're going to use drug substitution as a way of reducing harm, pot is a good choice. There are many medical marijuana organizations around the country that you can contact for specifics.

Caution Regarding the Long-Acting
Naltrexone Injection (brand name Vivitrol)

If you are going to have a medical procedure in the near future that might require opioid pain medications, **do not** take this long-acting drug. It will be difficult to get pain relief and may require a hospital visit to safely give you enough pain medications to override the opioid-blocking effects of the Vivitrol.

Abstinence

You have decided that you're done using. You may have added up the risks and harms and decided that the best move you can make is to stop using drugs altogether. They're expensive and illegal, and sometimes it's hard to know what you're getting. Or you've experi-

> Abstaining is sometimes the best harm reduction strategy. It's the quitting part that can be difficult!

enced a near fatal overdose (or several) and aren't willing to take that chance anymore. Some people simply find that abstaining is actually easier than trying to manage a drug-use pattern that is long-standing. Whatever the reason, you have several options, some limited by the laws in your state, but still options. If you want to quit, all of the preceding strategies can be used as steps toward quitting altogether if you so choose.

Quitting one or all of your drugs can be dangerous, or so difficult that you fail every time. This is when to consider "detox"—a supervised plan to detoxify your body without causing serious medical problems such as seizures, delirium tremens (DTs) from alcohol, dehydration, or cardiac problems. Many people detox themselves at home, alone or with a friend. If you already have medical issues, or if your level of physical dependence is pretty high, it might be safest (and most comfortable) to check yourself into a medical detoxification program. These often run from 5 to 10 days depending on the drug(s) you're using. Many are associated with treatment programs that are based on the 12 steps, so if you're not into that, make sure you let them know it's the medical detox you're looking for—period.

There are many options if you've decided to quit opioids, alcohol, or legal pills such as the antianxiety medications Klonopin, Xanax, and other benzodiazepines.

Cold Turkey

This means quitting with no substitutes, at home or in so-called nonmedical programs. For opioid withdrawal, you can take over-the-counter medications for diarrhea or muscle pain, but you're basically going to suffer a severe flu-like condition that will be at its worst by day 3 and pretty much be over by day 7. Some programs, called "social model detox centers," may offer some more comforts as well as counseling while you're going through it. Alcohol and antianxiety medications (benzos) *should not be quit cold turkey* if you've been using a lot over a period of months or years.

Medication-Assisted Detoxification

For drugs like heroin or codeine, this can refer to taking medicines that help reduce the severity of your symptoms but are not opioids. A better choice is opioid-assisted detox—either methadone or buprenorphine. Methadone can only be prescribed as part of a formal residential or outpatient program, but buprenorphine can be used at home under medical supervision. Most detox schedules are rapid, 3–10 days, and the relapse rate is high for this type of detox (up to 90%). A longer, slower reduction (3–6 months or longer) will probably give you a better chance of remaining abstinent.

For alcohol or benzos you could also consider talking to your primary care doctor to see if there are prescription medications that you could take at home to manage withdrawal symptoms. Long-acting benzodiazepines like Librium or Valium can be used for alcohol withdrawal and to detox slowly from the shorter-acting drugs like Xanax.

There are some non–FDA-approved detox treatments available as well. Ibogaine is being used with some success, but it is illegal in the United States. It does require careful monitoring, so if you choose to go this route, be careful to research the people and programs that are offering this treatment.

Medication-Assisted Abstinence

Opioid Substitution Treatment (or Maintenance)

As we mentioned before, this is a treatment, not a substitute "addiction" that gives you either methadone or buprenorphine at a dose that will prevent withdrawal and cravings. You will still be physically dependent on opioids, but you'd be amazed at how quickly you can begin to get your life back in order. You won't be looking for drugs or the money to buy them, overdosing, spending all of your time preoccupied by your use to the detriment of relationships, job, or school. Strangely enough, for all its success this can be a controversial treatment in the medical profession, and in some drug treatment programs they won't consider you "drug free" if you choose substitution treatment. Our opinion is that, at least for people who have a long history of using opioids (more than a year), substitution/maintenance is the best choice, at least for a while. Some people will do better staying on the medicine for life, while others can start a long, slow detox after a year or so—once you've got the rest of your life sorted out.

Some countries are now offering heroin maintenance therapy, which allows people to continue the use of their drug of choice without all of the legal and medical risks associated with unsupervised use. The research on this method is very encouraging, and its use extends as close to the United States as Canada, so we'll see if our country can get on board with it as we move in the direction of taking drug users' health seriously.

Alcohol Abstinence Medications

There is no substitute medication for alcohol. There are either medications that prevent you from using or medications that might help control cravings and the amount you use if you do slip up. Antabuse is the only medication that, as long as you use it, guarantees that you won't drink! It blocks an essential enzyme in the liver, and you'll get extremely ill if you drink while taking it. It can also kill you if mixed with too much alcohol.

Putting It All Together

Now you are ready to put it all together. You can change your drug use by making even small changes in the drug itself, in your mind-set, or in the setting in which you use. We have created a Drug, Set, Setting Goals form to identify each element that you would like to adjust. Use a separate form for each drug. The form is on page 164, or see the end of the Contents for information on printing out additional copies.

Here are three examples to give you some ideas about making changes in your drug, set, or setting:

Goal 1: Reduce the *amount* of pot that you smoke

1. Test your dose. Smoke a small amount, then wait to see whether you are satisfied with the effect. Excellent dosing suggestions can be found at *www.erowid.org/plants/cannabis/cannabis_dose.shtml*. (drug)

2. Don't smoke alone. (setting)

3. Don't keep pot in the house. (setting)

4. Buy stronger pot so you smoke less and/or begin to cook with it to avoid the harmful smoke. (drug)

5. Smoke only when you really need to. (set)

Maybe you could not smoke alone, but if it's there in your apartment, it's hard to resist. But if you *don't* keep pot in the house, you may not be able to find it when you need it, and that makes you feel anxious. So #1 isn't possible

My Drug, Set, Setting Goals

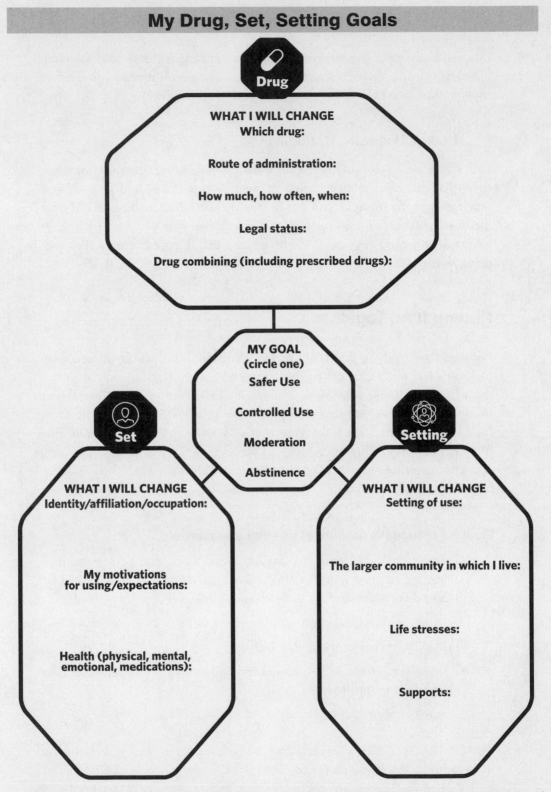

Drug

WHAT I WILL CHANGE
Which drug:

Route of administration:

How much, how often, when:

Legal status:

Drug combining (including prescribed drugs):

MY GOAL
(circle one)
Safer Use

Controlled Use

Moderation

Abstinence

Set

WHAT I WILL CHANGE
Identity/affiliation/occupation:

My motivations
for using/expectations:

Health (physical, mental,
emotional, medications):

Setting

WHAT I WILL CHANGE
Setting of use:

The larger community in which I live:

Life stresses:

Supports:

without #2, and #2 doesn't look like such a good idea to you right now. You are really in either the precontemplation (you can't even think about it) or the contemplation (it's a good idea if you could tolerate it, but you can't right now) stage of change regarding keeping yourself away from pot. With pot, amount is hard to quantify because there is the volume of marijuana itself as well as the amount of the active ingredient, THC. You might be able to reduce the amount of marijuana that you smoke simply by buying stronger pot. That way, you'll get high without using a lot and burning up your lungs. (On the other hand, if you smoke a lot partly because the activity is soothing, buying stronger pot will not reduce the amount! In that case, buy weaker stuff. You can smoke frequently but still be reducing the amount of THC you're taking in.) Perhaps buying stronger pot (#4) isn't financially practical or available where you live. That goes off the list for now as well because it's not manageable. You figure that you can tell when you really want to smoke alone—usually it's when you've had a stressful day at work or an argument with your girlfriend—as opposed to when you just do it out of habit, so #3 seems like a good place to start making a change. Now you need to make a plan for how to do that. Congratulations! You've arrived at the preparation stage.

Goal 2: Cut down on the *frequency* of your ecstasy use

1. Go to fewer parties. (setting)

2. Go to "sober" dances. (setting)

3. Switch to alcohol, which you don't actually like very much. (drug)

4. Develop some time-consuming hobbies. (set)

It's a great idea to go to fewer or to "sober" dance parties. It would sure stop you from using E. But it's your world, the dance scene. Not only do all your friends meet there, but you love to dance. It's your favorite way to move your body, especially since you aren't into sports. You're not even going to contemplate these ideas—talk about depression! That *would* be depressing, and you HATE it when your mother tells you she wants you to see a doctor because she thinks you're depressed. You consider alcohol. You definitely want a buzz when you're dancing, and a few beers would do it and be refreshing at the same time. On the other hand, you've heard that alcohol is more dangerous in the long run than E, so you're not sure it's a good switch. Still, you're contemplating it as a good possibility. Well, you do know that you get pretty moody, although you wouldn't admit it to anyone else. So you're reluctantly contemplating trying medication too.

Goal 3: Change the *route of administration* of heroin because you don't always shoot safe

1. Snort instead of shooting heroin. (drug)

2. Talk to other users at a needle exchange about your love of needles. (set)

3. Stay away from people who shoot. (setting) (but if you *do* end up injecting, please don't do it alone)

"No way," you say, "am I going to give up shooting." You know you're careless and share works. You know you have friends who have HIV and hepatitis C. But *nothing* beats the feeling of shooting dope. So forget that one. Nor are you going to leave your community and look for other people. Guess that means you are in the precontemplation stage for both of those ideas. Yet you think you *should* stop shooting. It would also help you taper off your dependence on the intense rush you get. All that's left is for you to just talk to people. Talk to people who have tried switching from needles to snorting and see if it really was that disappointing. Talk to people about needles. Really get into what you love about them. Talk until you can't talk anymore. Then see how you feel. Talking is a way of contemplating, too.

Working on these changes with someone else—whether or not he or she is a fellow user—is often very helpful. Be careful, though, not to make promises to other people. Make promises only to yourself and only about *trying* to change. The other person is a witness, a coach, a support—not a nag or a judge. He or she is *not supposed to hold you to your promises*!

Every time you come up with what seems to be a good idea about how to make healthier choices or changes in your drug use, do the same thing. Test out your idea according to how you feel about it, which will tell you the stage of change you are at. Trial and error will tell you best what works for you. You're the expert.

None of us likes to hear that practice makes perfect, but it actually does make a difference. You're trying to change important behaviors. Ways of being and relating to alcohol, drugs, people, and places get ingrained over time. Remember, change is slow. Start with the idea that seems the easiest to accomplish. Success increases our sense of being powerful and makes other changes easier. Or you might want to start with a change that will make a *huge* impact right away—like never driving if you're using or always cleaning your works. That way you're more likely to stay alive, healthy, and out of jail as you prepare to make other changes.

What's Next?

The next chapter is about helping you stay alive, healthy, and safe as you continue to use and to make your way through changing your drug use. It is about taking care of *you*—in the same way as anyone would take care of him- or herself.

As a drug user, you have as much right to safety, comfort, and enjoyment as anyone else, regardless of how you choose to get there.

9 Taking Care of Yourself While Still Using

Unconditional acceptance of each other is one of the greatest challenges we humans face. Few of us have experienced it consistently; the addict has never experienced it—least of all from himself.
—GABOR MATE, *In the Realm of Hungry Ghosts*

Taking care of yourself starts with believing that you deserve to be cared for. If you can accept being cared for, either literally with food and water, emotionally through good relationships, intellectually by stimulating work, projects, or entertainment, or socially by a caring community, it will be easier to change your relationship with drugs.

This chapter is devoted to *set*. Taking care of yourself means protecting your and others' safety; getting enough food, water, and sleep; managing your vulnerabilities—the things that drive your use; and surrounding yourself with people and things that make you feel OK. If you take care of yourself in these ways, your drug problems might change with far less effort than you anticipated. They might even just go away!

Taking Care of the Basics

Safety: Yours and Others'

Getting intoxicated can expose you to other risks. Besides the risks directly related to your use—overdose, disease transmission, liver disease, contaminated drugs, or bad trips—there are risks that can occur *while* you are using: accidents, violence, theft, unprotected sex, and arrest and incarceration. You might also be putting others at risk—your children, your husband, wife, partner, your grandparents, your neighbors, other people, especially if you're driving drunk or impaired by other drugs.

168

Violence and Accidents

It is hard to overstate the impact of alcohol on violence. Alcohol is a factor in 40% of all violent crimes today, according to the Department of Justice. More than any illegal drug, alcohol was found to be closely associated with violent crimes, including murder, rape, assault, and child and spousal abuse. About half of all homicides and assaults are committed when the offender, victim, or both have been drinking, and alcohol is often a factor in violence where the attacker and the victim know each other. Other drugs are sometimes associated with violence as well, but the picture is often complicated by the fact that these drugs are illegal. For example, there is a clear association between drugs and violence, but much of it is related to drug dealing, turf wars, and the dangers of sex work rather than interpersonal violence due to being high. Drugs such as PCP and amphetamines have been shown to increase the risk for interpersonal violence.

As for accidents, it is commonly known that alcohol leads to falls, motor vehicle crashes, and drowning. Stimulant drugs can encourage high-risk behaviors that result in injury (climbing towers, playing chicken with an oncoming train). Drugs that cause sedation or motor control problems can result in falls and other traumatic injuries.

> *Alcohol is consistently shown to be a risk factor for aggression, including in a recent laboratory study.*

Date Rape and Party Rape

Almost 100,000 college students report an alcohol-related sexual assault each year. If you are going to drink and party, or use other drugs, especially sedating drugs like GHB or pills (which are usually either pain medications or benzos), take a few precautions. Watch your drinks to make sure no one is

Two-thirds of victims who were attacked by a current or former intimate partner reported that alcohol had been involved.

- Nearly 4 in 10 child victimizers reported that they had been drinking at the time of the abuse.

- A 1999 study by the National Center on Addiction and Substance Abuse found that children of substance-misusing parents were almost three times more likely to be abused and more than four times likelier to be neglected than children of parents who did not misuse substances.

adding anything. If you are partying with men (regardless of your gender), stay conscious or be with a friend who is. We know that getting obliterated is sometimes the point. Do it when you aren't with people who can overpower and hurt you. Know what you are taking—this can be hard at a party, but do your best. Get assertiveness training. Learn self-defense.

If you are the victim of assault while partying, it doesn't matter that you are a drinker or drug user. You have the right not to be harmed! Know this, remind yourself of this. Think about whether your choice of friends and intimate partners is putting you at risk. Work with a therapist who can help you improve your self-esteem and change how you choose partners. Find people who think you're wonderful and treat you well. If you don't know any, decide to start looking.

> Never forget: You have the right not to be harmed!

This is a time to do a decisional balance (see Chapter 7). Figure out which of your risks is most dangerous. For example, are you likely to drink too much and not have a designated driver? Or are you more likely to down a whole handful of pills, *not* test the strength of your shot, or drink too fast and end up semiconscious and thus more likely to fall prey to sexual aggression? The bottom line is: if you're going to get wasted, have someone around to steer you out of harm's way, not someone who will take advantage of your altered state.

Sex Work and Safety

People don't talk much about sex work other than to say that it is illegal and people who do it are criminals (or worse). But many women, and a smaller but significant number of men, earn a living by providing sexual services for a fee. This work carries with it the multiple harms of stigma, arrest and incarceration, and the threat of physical violence. To add insult to injury,

Are You Putting Yourself or Others at Risk?

If the kids wake up sick in the middle of the night . . . can you wake up to help them?

Buzzed driving is . . . buzzed driving (whether alcohol, pills, weed, or speed).

Do you have a stash of condoms, and do you use them?

few health care workers pay attention to the unique needs of sex workers. If you are part of, or on the fringes of, this industry, you know that alcohol and drugs play a big part in the scene and in the work. Hopefully, this book will speak to you and give you tools that you can use in negotiating your contracts with your customers. What most people don't know is that, despite the hazards of sex work, there is also a strong community. Find it! Being alone in this work is not good for your emotional or physical well-being. A good health and safety resource for sex workers has been written by the staff of St. James Infirmary (in San Francisco). You can download it for free at *www.stjamesinfirmary.org.*

Arrest and Incarceration

Being in jail or prison is very bad for your health. The dangers of gang violence and sexual assault, poor sleep, inadequate access to natural light, lack of exercise, inadequate medical and mental health treatment, and very bad food all have a negative impact on your physical and mental health. We repeat the words of Ethan Nadelmann: More harm has been done by the War on Drugs than was ever done by drug use. African Americans and Latinos are at highest risk of being stopped and frisked, arrested, charged with a drug-related crime, and incarcerated. People who are homeless, whose living room is on the streets, are also at high risk. All that said, it is very important to avoid arrest. See the box on the next page for help in knowing your legal rights.

Harm reduction alert: When you leave jail or prison (or a drug treatment program), your risk of overdose on certain drugs increases because your tolerance has decreased. (It takes less to get you high.) *If you were dependent on opioids before you went in and you are going to return to using, don't use as much when you come out.* You have to build up your tolerance again, so take it slow. Lower your dose and test your shot.

And Now Some Advice from Your Harm Reduction Mothers

You might have heard of Abraham Maslow's "hierarchy of needs." It begins with humans' basic survival needs and evolves to our need to "self-actualize," or achieve our full potential. In other words, if one is starving, it is hard to think of anything but food. People who use and misuse alcohol and other drugs have additional needs because of the physical, psychological, social, and environmental impacts of intoxicating substances. So while the following tips might seem somewhat obvious from a basic health perspective, they may be particularly important for you.

Know Your Rights

If you are a user of illegal drugs, or if you are a user of alcohol who gets into trouble—DUI, drug test at work, domestic violence—you have rights. While no one has the right to harm other people, your legal rights still need to be protected and respected. The Drug Policy Alliance maintains an up-to-date website with information on the current drug laws in each state. Go to *www.drugpolicy.org/drug-laws-criminal-justice-system-and-you*. Some highlights include information on:

- Where drugs are a misdemeanor or a felony

- Illegal search and seizure

- Court-mandated AA (which is unconstitutional)

- DUI—driver's license and professional license suspensions

- Laws regarding fetal drug exposure by pregnant women

- Drug testing

- Naloxone (it can now be distributed over the counter in pharmacies)

- Over-the-counter sale of needles

- Good Samaritan laws protecting drug users who call 911 during a drug-related medical emergency

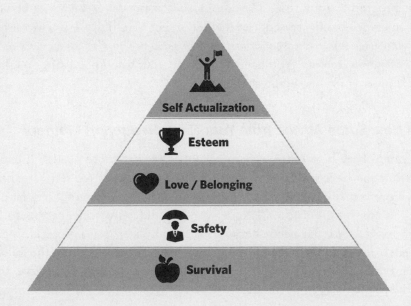

Breathe. Breathe air that is fresh and makes you feel good. Take a breath of oxygen between hits of inhalable drugs. Focus on your breathing when you are anxious—slow it down and count your breaths.

Drink your water. Besides all the well-known reasons to drink water, being dehydrated poses an additional problem for drug users. People who smoke cigarettes, drink alcohol, coffee, or tea, or use drugs like ecstasy and speed that raise heart rate, blood pressure, and body temperature should drink more water than others. Your kidneys will thank you.

Eat. First of all, just eat. Then worry about *what* you're eating. If you want to moderate the effects of your drugs or stabilize your blood sugar as you intoxicate your mind, eat before you drink or use. Finally, find a website whose advice about food you appreciate and that doesn't make you feel hopeless about ever maintaining a virtuous nutrition program.

Sleep. All animals need sleep. Some of us need less, some more. Sleep is essential to both physical and mental health. The less you sleep, the lower your resistance to illness. Not getting enough sleep can exacerbate depression and anxiety. Sleep deprivation can cause everything from garden-variety exhaustion, difficulty thinking, or irritability to depression, anxiety, and feeling downright crazy. Sleeplessness is also a *symptom* of depression and anxiety. Although many people use alcohol and other drugs to get to sleep, alcohol disrupts the sleep cycle and stimulants stop it altogether. (Which is sometimes the point!)

So sleep. Nap in the afternoon. Nap at your desk at lunchtime. Nap in the morning after you take the kids to school or after the early shift is over. Talk to your doctor if you're having trouble sleeping. Find a doctor who won't refuse you sleep aids because you are a drinker or drug user. If that's hard, there are many over-the-counter and natural remedies—not to mention chamomile tea, a couple of restorative yoga poses, or a meditation tape.

Stay warm. There's a reason the words *cold* and *lonely* often appear in the same sentence. When you're cold, it feels like the only thing to do is to curl into yourself, shut your eyes, and hope it will go away. There is even a research study that showed that people who were socially isolated actually felt colder than those in a control group. Alcohol feels like it warms you because it stimulates the blood vessels near the surface of your skin to expand, but it doesn't really. Stimulants do actually raise body temperature. Opioids are often described as a warm blanket. Just as *cold* and *lonely* are linked, so are *warmth* and *comfort*. So stay warm—literally—and find comfort where you can. Once you are warm and comfortable, you might find that you use differently.

Find love. People, like all animals, need closeness and connection as much

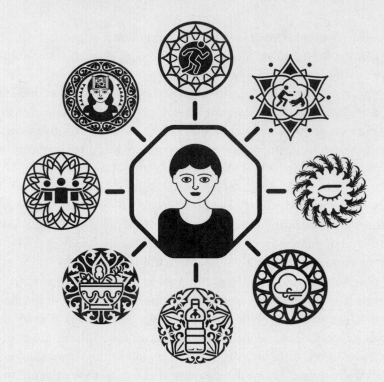

as anything else. We need love. Animals who do not have connection and love fail to thrive. We become anxious and depressed. Some of us become self-destructive. If you are alienated from people, if you fear relationships, hang out with an animal. It will help to keep you alive.

Taking Care of the Things That Drive Your Use

We've talked a lot in this book about how important it is to understand *why* you use if you're going to change your use and reduce its harm. When you know what's driving your use, you can consider other ways to manage it that might help.

Pain

The bottom line is that you need to get adequate medications, alternative treatments, or both.

One of the most underrecognized phenomena that drug users experience is physical pain. Pain is undertreated in general in the United States—and we're not just talking about people who have been identified as "addicts."

We are talking about postsurgical patients, accident victims, and, most of all, people in chronic pain. Pain is so undertreated that the American Medical Association has written policy guidelines on the appropriate treatment of pain, and in 1997 the State of California passed a bill detailing the rights of patients with intractable pain to receive adequate treatment.

As we write this book, Americans are experiencing high rates of overdose on opioid medications. The DEA is scrutinizing doctors' prescriptions for pain medication, which in turn is causing doctors to cut back on pain prescriptions. If you've been labeled an "addict," you'll have a hard time getting adequate help with pain management. Surely it is not coincidental that we have seen a fourfold increase in heroin use in the last 10 years. People start with prescribed medicines, run out of pills and/or money, and turn to street heroin, with all of the potential harms of hygiene and overdose.

Most people who use prescribed opioids for pain relief do *not* misuse them; they take them as prescribed. Of the people who take more than prescribed, we would be willing to wager that they do so because they have not been prescribed enough to manage their pain. This phenomenon is called *pseudo-addiction*. It does not come with the psychological compulsion that characterizes "addiction" or compulsive drug use. It comes from undertreated pain. Let's say you break your leg and have surgery to repair it. Your doctor prescribes an opioid pain medicine and instructs you to take one every 4 to 6 hours. But the doctor wrote the prescription so that at the pharmacy you get only enough pills to take one every 6 hours, not every 4 hours! It turns out each dose wears off at the 4-hour point, so you take another. Now you're going to run out before you can get a refill. So you call in for another prescription and get labeled as a pill seeker, which *you are*! But you're not looking to get high; you're seeking an adequate dose of your medicine.

> Most people who use prescribed opioids for pain relief do *not* misuse them.

The best way to start the process of getting adequate care for pain is to find a pain management clinic or pain specialist. Most will use at least some additional nonmedical treatments, such as meditation or acupuncture. Most will prescribe some medications. Some might prescribe enough to take care of all your pain management needs.

Stress, Trauma, and Posttraumatic Stress

Stress is pressure. The right amount provides energy. Too little and we are passive. Too much and we might break. Both challenging *and* happy events are stressful: the death of a child or a spouse, getting divorced, the birth of a child, moving, losing your home, having a heart attack, changing jobs, being promoted, or getting fired. Less dramatic stresses include graduating from high school or college, losing your bicycle, or breaking a leg.

How much stress is too much is individual to each person—it depends on your resilience and on the other things going on in your life. Too much stress can make you vulnerable to catching a cold, losing your keys, yelling at your partner or kids, falling down the stairs, drinking more alcohol, or using more drugs. Stress compromises your immune system and lowers your resistance to illness and accidents. Stressful experiences, whether happy or sad, have one thing in common: they all involve loss or change.

> Stress can come from positive as well as negative experiences.

Too much stress leads to *emotional distress.* When we say, "I'm beside myself!" or "I can't take it anymore!" we are communicating emotional distress. Changing your drug use can arouse emotional distress too. If you've quit, if you're cutting down, or if you're changing how, where, or when you use, you'll probably notice yourself experiencing strong anger, anxiety, or even elation. Don't be surprised if you cut down on your pot smoking for a month and, all of a sudden, *wham*! You're feeling really sad, crying at the least little thing, and have no idea why.

Regardless of the source, what we need at such times is to be soothed, to be reassured and comforted. It's the feeling we get when someone rubs our back or strokes our head and says, "Shhhh, everything's going to be all right now." Ideally, as we grow up, we develop the same ability to soothe ourselves. This is called *self-soothing*. Self-soothing is one of the things that helps humans "regulate" our emotions. Emotion regulation refers to the ability to experience a full range of feelings in response to people or events, to tolerate emotional arousal, to react both spontaneously and with restraint to events and to other people, and to recover one's equilibrium after emotionally wrenching experiences.

People who have had too much stress have difficulty soothing themselves. Edward Khantzian, who developed the self-medication hypothesis

> Difficulty managing strong emotions (including the inability to soothe themselves) is one of the core issues that cause some people to self-medicate with substances.

we introduced in Chapter 4, believes that difficulty managing strong emotions (including the inability to soothe themselves) is one of the core issues that cause some people to self-medicate with substances. Often these are the people whose stress has crossed the line into *trauma*.

Trauma refers to *any experience* that (1) is beyond the realm of normal and expected human experience; (2) involves actual or threatened death or injury, either to oneself or others; (3) causes fear or horror and intense physical or emotional distress; and (4) overwhelms one's ability to cope, even for a short time. Traumatic events include *natural disasters* such as earthquakes, fires, or famine; *community or national events* like war or genocide; the *ongoing effects* of racism; *family circumstances* such as hunger and poverty, domestic violence, child abuse or neglect, or the death of a parent, sibling, or child; and *personal experiences* such as rape, imprisonment, accident, or medical illness. Some people heal from such experiences: they manage to get through life without major disruption to their ability to work, love, and laugh. Unfortunately, others develop symptoms of posttraumatic stress disorder (PTSD). As we described in Chapter 4, people with a lot of childhood trauma use drugs at far higher rates than anyone else. PTSD is a complex neurobiological and psychological response to trauma that emerges after the experience is over. Symptoms include those listed in the box below.

> Trauma and drug use go hand in hand.

Sometimes trauma impacts all aspects of a person's life—how we reacted to trauma becomes part of who we are. We become people who do not trust, are prone to guilt and shame, and get into relationships that repeat the very experiences that hurt us in the first place. This is called developmental trauma. When we are affected to this extent, it is time to consider therapy.

Symptoms of PTSD

- *Reexperiencing*: intrusive thoughts, flashbacks, or nightmares.

- *Avoidance*: avoiding people, places, or things associated with the trauma.

- *Emotional numbness*: loss of interest and detachment.

- *Hyperarousal*: hypervigilance, anxiety, anger, difficulty falling asleep, or exaggerated startle response.

- *Psychological and emotional distress*: depression, guilt, and shame; loss of meaning, loss of faith, cynicism; damage to one's identity and self-esteem.

- *Reenactment*: courting danger in high-risk sports or hobbies or repeatedly getting into violent relationships, either as a victim or as a perpetrator.

Drugs can relieve tension, soothe distress, and distract from the demons that haunt us. We're not stupid—we don't generally use drugs to be self-destructive. We use them for reasons, very good ones. And they work! Until they don't. So, as you go about changing your relationship with drugs, or not, you'll need to take care of your stress, your distress, and your traumatic symptoms, if you have them, so you don't catch cold (or worse), fall down the stairs (or worse), or lose your keys (or worse).

Taking Care of Stress and Trauma

There are many formal and informal stress reduction techniques, available on hundreds of websites and in thousands of books. Alan Marlatt, the late harm reduction researcher, wrote an excellent book on mindfulness and relapse prevention. Formal stress reduction techniques include things like mindfulness meditation, massage, and breathing exercises. Or simply take a long hot shower, wrap yourself up in your favorite sweatshirt, sit in bed reading the sports section, or eat some mashed potatoes or other "comfort food." A therapy model specially designed to help people manage emotions and behavior is dialectical behavior therapy (DBT). Cognitive-behavioral therapy (CBT) focuses on dispelling false beliefs and toxic thoughts so that one becomes more emotionally balanced. On the facing page is a short self-care guide developed with a colleague who works in a high-stress environment.

For those of you who need to move, yoga, martial arts, walking, or more strenuous physical exercise in which you break a sweat and discharge some of the built-up tension might work well. Singing in the car or the shower is also good, as is standing under a noisy, well-trafficked bridge (to muffle the noise) and shouting out your frustrations.

Many therapies exist to treat posttraumatic stress—from talking psychotherapies to medicines to body-oriented therapies. An excellent resource is the Trauma Center (*www.traumacenter.org*), founded by Dr. Bessel van der Kolk, one of the foremost trauma researchers in the world. His center develops and researches the therapeutic effectiveness of activities like choral singing, "trauma drama," and trauma-sensitive yoga.

Co-occurring Problems

As we discussed in Chapter 4, co-occurring psychiatric and emotional disorders are the rule for drug users, not the exception. But you may not realize just how your drug use is connected to your symptoms of depression or anxiety or hearing voices. You know that you sleep better if you drink or that

> ### Self-Care Reminders
>
> <u>Understand yourself</u>
> Ask yourself, "What's the matter?"
> Truly listen to the answer
> Give yourself permission to be upset—it's really OK
> <u>Self-regulate</u>
> Walk around the block
> Splash water on your face
> Find someone to talk to . . .
> . . . or cry with
> Drink tea or ice-cold water
> Hold something cold
> Breathe
> Take deep, slow breaths
> Say "Wow" with a deep breath
> Laugh
> *Try to laugh each day. Laughter is an amazing way to release tension.*
> <u>Debrief</u>
> Vent
> Reflect on what went well
> Plan for next time
>
> ─────────────
> Thanks to Melanie Garner at the Tenderloin Housing Clinic for putting together this guide.

you're not nearly as anxious after shooting heroin. But you might not realize that when you can't get to sleep the night after drinking, it might actually be *because* of the drinking you did yesterday! Or that your anxiety might actually be a sign of withdrawal from the heroin that you didn't use today. Drug use and your symptoms are related in very complicated ways, ways that may not make sense to you unless you really study your experience. Take another look at the "Harms Minus the Hysteria" section in Chapter 3 and see if your situation is mentioned. Then revisit your own harms and benefits worksheet to see if you might have missed some connections. Keeping a record of how and what you feel before and after using will give you some hints as to drug effects that you just didn't know were making things worse in the long run even though they help in the short run.

Whether you are using stimulants to treat ADHD, cigarettes for schizo-phrenia, alcohol or pot or opioids for PTSD, pot for anxiety, alcohol for depression, or any of the dozens of other ways to self-medicate, you might need professional help to manage the symptoms you experience. The tips in this chapter, while they may help to calm you and help you feel healthier, might not be enough to take care of the full complexity of your issues.

If you are having trouble managing your substance use, and you are concerned about your mental and emotional health, seek consultation from a mental health professional, preferably one who is friendly to the principles of harm reduction, even if not formally a harm reduction therapist or doctor. If that is not possible, just find a therapist you can talk to about all of your feelings and symptoms. Chapter 11 will give you more guidance about finding help.

Impulsiveness

Most people who have problems with alcohol or other drugs have gotten into the habit of acting on their feelings rather than just feeling them. When they feel bad, they have to *do* something. Solution: get buzzed, drunk, or high—anything to avoid those feelings. Impulse is the thing we are acting on when we experience the triggers and cravings that we talked about in Chapter 8. Here are some alternatives:

Build Emotional Muscle

There are several ways to get used to feelings so that you don't have to *do* something immediately. The main idea is to *stop*! Put some distance between your urge to do something and actually doing it. Our colleague Andrew Tatarsky, a harm reduction therapist in New York, talks about "creating space between the impulse and the action." What he means is stopping and paying attention to the impulse and tracking it back to the event or the feeling that preceded it. In so doing, you might develop other ideas about how to respond to the event or feeling that impelled you to act.

Practice is at the heart of any method. Just as exercise builds physical muscle, using your feelings will also increase your tolerance, stamina, and "emotional muscle" so that you will be less vulnerable to the stresses of being human. But delaying gratification is a skill that also comes with practice. Sometimes we just have to wait to get what we want.

Count. Remember being told as a kid that you should count to 10 when you were mad before you did or said anything, so that you didn't hit somebody, say mean things, or have a tantrum? Well, it's the same idea now. Just count and stay as still as you can. We all forget that feelings, even the strongest ones, change, maybe even evaporate. Each time you feel yourself

Building Emotional Muscle

STOP and count

WAIT—distract yourself

FOCUS—surf the urge

getting really sad or angry or frustrated, *count.* If you get to 3 and then can't take it anymore, that's fine. Get yourself to 3 and then scream, fall apart, whatever. Next time, maybe you can get to 5 or 10. Keep increasing the time between feeling something and taking an action until you can sit with most feelings, either until they pass (most do) or until you can plan what you want to do.

Distract yourself. Counting is about holding it in rather than exploding. Some drugs, like heroin or pot, help you hold things in. Others, like alcohol, help you let them out. Often you end up letting things out that you regret the next day. If you can't sit still, can't hold it in, go ahead and let it out. But try something besides alcohol or slamming drugs. Run, walk, slam a door, sing along to a really loud song. But try not to yell at your partner, kick the dog, or slam your fist into a wall.

If you are a quiet sort of person, read, do the *I Ching,* pray, or meditate. If you are drawn to stimulants, you will need stimulation. Movies, video games (which can, of course, become an obsession in themselves), playing or watching fast or high-risk sports, things that both de-stress you and make you feel alive.

Surf the urge. A slightly more difficult skill is sometimes referred to as *urge surfing,* introduced in Chapter 8—staying still and *concentrating* on the urge rather than trying to avoid it. In the ocean, you can't escape the wave, you have to understand it and ride it. An urge or a craving lasts for about 20 minutes. Learn what the urge really is: a desperate need to run away from whatever it is you're feeling, a strong desire for a different feeling or sensation, or a wish to be part of a group or scene.

Taking Care of Your Surroundings (Your Setting)

Your Environment

Remember Rat Park and the rats who used far less morphine when they were in a more natural environment that had the things rats like, including other rats. If you live in an unsafe or unfriendly environment, find a place that makes you feel welcome and calm—café, beach, woods, friend's house, needle exchange program or supervised injection facility, political gathering, favorite bar (ask the bartender to hold your keys and give you the evil eye when you have had enough).

- Put *things* in your environment that serve as a touchstone and remind you of who you are at your core. Surround yourself with things that you like to look at.

- Do things that ground you—wash the dishes, clean the bathroom, weed or plant the garden, play cards, or cook.

- Pay attention to your surroundings—really look around. Whether you are looking at something you like or something you hate, pay attention to it. Study it. Think about what you like or dislike about it. Whatever it is, it will change your perspective on other things— your wife, your kids, your job, or your drugs—when you return your attention to them.

Your People

Remember self-determination theory—good relationships are good for your motivation, your sense of well-being, and your health. So find life-affirming people, people who nurture your self-esteem. Hang around people who:

- Don't judge

- Like you

- Will tuck you in at night when you have messed up

- Are outside of your drug-using community and can give you other perspectives—not even on you, but on life, on politics, on baseball, on anything that can take you outside of yourself. They can be old people who knew you when you weren't so down and out. Or they can be new people. What is important is that they *not* talk to you about drugs.

Do something for them too. Get outside of your needs and your sorrows. Give them flowers, cook them a meal, pick up their kids from school. It will get you outside of yourself. And that will help you to gain perspective on your relationship with drugs and whether it is really essential to who you are and how you live.

The Big Picture

Your Values

Researchers in motivation have found that focusing on what you value, what is important to you, can ground you and help steer your course. Your values are your core beliefs, the beliefs that guide your decisions and your life. Values are much the same as morals or ethics. Values include things like the Golden Rule (treat others as you would have them treat you), generosity, and tolerance.

Some people derive their values from formal spiritual or religious practices—Christianity, Judaism, Islam, Buddhism, or polytheistic, nature-based, or feminine-based practices. Others draw their values from political perspectives—whether conservative, liberal, socialist, or libertarian. Some take their values from philosophers or great writers, and others from observations of the natural world. Harm reduction also has a set of values, values that are grounded in human rights and freedom from harm; see the box on the next page.

Your Mind: Expand Your Horizons

Drugs often isolate people from the non-drug-using world and from the kinds of mental stimulation offered by getting involved with other people, political issues, reading, and cultural developments in music, art, theater, or movies. For some people, working too hard is part of that isolation. For others, the isolation comes from being bored and having too little to do. One of the major contributions of 12-step groups is that they get people out of the house and involved with others. If you don't like 12-step programs, however, you won't get that benefit. If you don't want to join a group or program, it might be very useful to you—and to the world of which you are a citizen—to get involved in a cause that you can support. Read the paper, go to movies, go to rallies, write letters to Congress about something that is important to you, defend the rights of drug users to have equal access to health care, whatever suits you. The important point is to

> Your drug use does *not* strip you of your membership in the human race, and we all need and will benefit from your involvement!

> # The Core Values of Harm Reduction
>
> - *Understanding.* Understand your choices and the things you have done in your life so far. Knowing *why* you use is essential to figuring out what to do about it.
>
> - *Acceptance.* Accept yourself and your choices and receive acceptance from others. Don't minimize the damage you might have done, but appreciate that you have done your best to survive and look for the strengths, the humor, and the cleverness in your efforts.
>
> - *Compassion.* Guilt is paralyzing, and you must forgive yourself, and hopefully be forgiven, for the damage you have done in order to move forward in your quest to find solutions.
>
> - *Kindness.* Be kind to yourself and hang around people who are kind to you.
>
> - *Connection.* Attachment—to Chivas Regal, the crack pipe, weed—can be replaced by, or exist alongside, connection to other people.
>
> - *Freedom to choose.* By this we do not mean independence from the needs and wants of others. We mean freedom from the punitive restrictions of others. We mean autonomy—the right and the opportunity to have a hand in the direction of your life.

remember that you *do* belong in the world. Your drug use does *not* strip you of your membership in the human race, and we all need and will benefit from your involvement!

Fun and Joy

If your alcohol or drug use has gotten out of hand, chances are you're not having as much fun as you used to. Using takes a lot of time, money, and worry and doesn't give back as much as it did at first. This leaves you without much fun in your life. Switching drugs is probably not the answer to this particular problem. Let's try another tack. Can you remember a time in your life when you enjoyed something? Watching the Three Stooges, walking on the beach, swimming in the river, sleeping in the sun, throwing a football or a baseball, digging in the garden, writing poetry? *That* is what life is about. Drugs are fun too, but if they have gotten in the way of joy, they are limiting your engagement in life. And if you don't have fun, quitting or changing your drugs is going to be a grind. So start doing something that gives you joy. Trying to get control of a drug or alcohol problem is not fun, so it's important that you *not* be working at it all the time!

What's Next?

This chapter has been all about how focusing on yourself apart from your drugs will help you manage your drug use. We hope that you have been comforted and inspired by it.

The working section of this book is over. Now it's time to reflect on how you are doing, seek help if you need it, and communicate with others. How can you tell if your harm reduction plan is working for you? Since we keep saying that it's complicated, in the next chapter we'll give you a guide to assess how well this is working for you.

> You can take care of yourself in many different ways, in any particular order, or all at the same time. It's entirely up to you.
>
> The more nurtured you are, the better your chances of managing your drug use.
>
> You can be a drug user *and* be a part of life.

10 How Can I Tell If Harm Reduction Is Working?

In other words, 80% of something is better than 100% of nothing.
    —ALEX WODAK, Australian drug policy
    reformer and harm reduction leader

Better is better.
    —KEN ANDERSON, founder of the
    HAMS Network

Is harm reduction working? You can tell by the fact that you are still reading this book! Nevertheless, it is a question that we are asked often. The dominant focus on abstinence as the most important measure of success and suspicion about harm reduction, at least as of 2017, makes it hard to feel confident that harm reduction is working. Dr. Wodak, a harm reduction pioneer and longtime drug policy reformer in Australia, is telling us in the statement above that harm reduction works when we set realistic and achievable goals. If our goals are unachievable, we get nowhere. If they are realistic, we make progress. This is why Lance Dodes, in his book *The Sober Truth,* estimates the success rate of AA at about 7%. Unrealistic goals are also why 40% of people say they don't go to substance use treatment programs (because they are not ready to commit to abstinence), why the completion rate of programs is 30–50%, and why fewer than 50% of people achieve the stated goals of the programs when they do finish.

Substance use treatment programs increasingly report harm reduction *outcomes,* despite the fact that they do not offer clients harm reduction *options.* For example, they report that drug treatment completion lowers the rate of loss of employment, improves family relationships, and results in fewer drug/alcohol using days. *Note they do not say* abstinence. Harm reduction data make the programs look more successful. If treatment programs are more successful when they measure themselves according to harm reduction standards, it is highly likely that you will be more successful using these standards too.

Just like these programs, most people in your life don't accept harm reduction as a way out of drug problems. The pressure is to get "clean and sober." Only then can your friends, family, or coworkers be reassured that you *got* it. No doubt that voice lives somewhere in your head too. Our goal in this chapter is to show you what "working" looks like—to reassure you that if you are doing certain things at different stages, then you are doing exactly what you need to do to make lasting changes. We offer some fairly detailed examples of how different people have made harm reduction work. Finally, we give you a chart that you can use to track your work and your progress.

First let's define what *working* means. Harm reduction works for different people in different ways. It works in smaller ways, like switching from smoking joints to vaporizing, to very big ways, like quitting pot altogether. When measuring improvement in harm reduction practice, you should be both *generous* and *realistic*. If you're thinking of giving up harm reduction because you don't see any improvement, be generous with yourself: Have things gotten any worse? Have you hurt or killed anyone? If the answer to both of these questions is "no" and you're still alive, harm reduction is probably working. In other words, if things were going downhill and you stopped the downhill slide, that's progress. Not getting worse might have saved someone's life.

On the other hand, if learning about harm reduction ends up making you so relaxed that you write off everybody's worries about you as drug hysteria, check again. Be realistic. Was there anything that *you* were worried about that needs attention? The likelihood is that, since you are still reading this book, you are taking your relationship with drugs seriously, have an appropriate level of concern, and have not climbed into a hole with your favorite drug to wait out the storm.

As we said in Chapter 6, one of the biggest reasons we don't make changes that we intended is that we are astonished at how much effort it takes and how long we have to put in that effort. Over time, we slow down (or even quit trying to change). This is just reality and not a measure of your character, your honesty, or even your motivation. Because of the hype that harm reduction "lets" people use, most people don't realize that harm reduction is a lot of work, especially if you're trying to manage a drug that had been out of control. Quitting would probably be easier! But if you aren't making the changes that you want, check yourself again and see if you really are putting effort into it. If not, revisit your decisional balance to make sure

> When in doubt about how your harm reduction efforts are working, review your plan and make sure it was realistic to begin with.

you really made a decision to change and aren't still sitting on the fence. Remember why you started this process in the first place. Get reenergized and reinspired. Then revisit your plan. Make sure it is realistic.

If you're still not sure what it means for harm reduction to be working, take a look at the box on the facing page.

What "Working" Looks Like: Cheryl, Tyler, and Ruben

In this section, we will finish telling you how Cheryl, Tyler, and Ruben made harm reduction work for them.

Cheryl

Cheryl's situation shows how harm reduction can work simultaneously with many life issues, even though substances are playing a large part in the problems she faces. Cheryl had thought about therapy for a while but didn't want a therapist who would focus on her drinking and tell her to go to AA. She read a newspaper article about moderate drinking as an alternative to AA and abstinence. She contacted us and began treatment.

Months 1–2: In the beginning, it took some coaxing to help Cheryl realize that she didn't have to reveal her entire life history to begin therapy with us. We encouraged her start with her current situation. We assessed that, while she was drinking more than is healthy, she was not in any imminent danger. She didn't drive after drinking, she didn't experience blackouts, and she didn't put herself in dangerous social situations.

Months 3–4: Cheryl worked on the interaction between her job stress and her drinking. This was a more straightforward problem and could be worked on behaviorally without much exploration of underlying issues. Too often, people with histories of trauma are encouraged to begin with the story of their abuse. But this tends to make people worse by activating the very feelings that they are trying to manage by using drugs! Instead, we helped Cheryl identify the parts of her job that were causing stress, then separate what she might have some control over and what she would have to learn to cope with. She developed stress reduction plans such as meditation and walks with friends after work instead of hitting happy hour. She also began

Harm reduction is working if either or both of the following are happening:

You are making any positive change!

> Keeping naloxone on hand . . . switching from vodka to beer . . . eating before you drink . . . drinking water before you drink, and during, and after . . . turning Friday night into movie night so you don't start partying until Saturday . . . turning one weekend a month into a family visit . . . switching from a pipe to a vaporizer . . . from cigarettes to e-cigarettes . . . hooking up with a needle exchange program . . . using a sleep aid besides alcohol . . . quitting partying at noon on Sunday, or arranging a late start on Mondays . . . trying doctor-prescribed rather than self-prescribed medication for depression, bipolar disorder, or anxiety.

> *. . . and/or following a* process *of change.*

If you . . .

> . . . are getting hassled by other people and are listening to at least one of them

> . . . have learned something new about the harms that might come from your use

> . . . are reflecting on your relationship with one of your drugs

> . . . have set a goal

> . . . are making a plan

> . . . have changed *something*

> . . . are building parts of your life that do not involve drugs

> . . . have achieved your goals and are *not* thinking about drugs

> . . . *then harm reduction is working.*

If you are . . .

listening	learning	reflecting
deciding	planning	experimenting
sticking it	building up other parts of your life	over it

. . . you are doing exactly what you need to do. You're putting effort into doing less harm to yourself and others. You don't have to be all finished. You don't have to quit using unless you decide to. You can take breaks. You get to decide how much work is the right amount. And you get to choose which harmful effects you want to work on based on their impact on your life. Remember, "any positive change" is all we humans can expect of ourselves.

to identify the things that she couldn't control—her schedule and her boss's moods. We helped her come up with some stock phrases to help her keep her cool in these situations. Her favorite one was "It's not my circus, and those aren't my monkeys." With this phrase, she could separate herself from the chaos around her and just get on with her own work.

Months 5–7: Cheryl got down to discussing her alcohol use. Now that she felt like she had some tools to cope with stress, the thought of cutting down on her drinking didn't seem so daunting. We asked her to keep a log of when, where, and how much she drank, and what she was feeling. With this specific information we helped her identify triggers and create alternate strategies. She then set a goal: no more than two glasses of wine, and not more than 3 nights a week. She was able to successfully keep her drinking to two glasses of wine but continued to drink most every night. She felt frustrated and like a failure for not doing "better." We reminded her that this was a big change already and maybe she needed time to adjust to the lower quantity before tackling the frequency. During this time, she did not increase her Vicodin use. She was not ready to address it though.

Months 8–12: Cheryl kept her drinking at two glasses and was often successful at not drinking every night. When she began a new relationship, she and we decided that it was time to tackle the more difficult issue of drinking to overcome the traumatic response she had to sexual relationships. The therapy shifted focus to decreasing her stress response to sex, learning to stop the anticipatory anxiety that she experienced before an upcoming date, and giving herself "time-outs"—canceling plans or stopping a sexual encounter if she didn't feel relaxed. She decided not to drink at all for 6 months to really learn how to manage her anxieties without alcohol. Again, her Vicodin use remained stable.

Months 13–18: Cheryl continued to work on relationship issues with much success. She had maintained a relationship with the "perfect man" for almost a year and was still not drinking. She decided that alcohol would never be a regular part of her life but reserved the right to drink on celebratory occasions. At this point, feeling secure in her drinking plan, Cheryl declared that she was ready to tackle her Vicodin habit. She engaged in somatic therapy with a trauma specialist which helped to reduce dramatically her trauma response to sexual intimacy. Within 3 months she had quit altogether.

Tyler

Tyler kept thinking about how his life didn't compare very well with his friends' lives. He was just marking time, and the negative consequences of his alcohol and speed use were adding up. He looked around online for a while, but the idea of rehab seemed extreme. He didn't feel "addicted" to alcohol or speed; he just partied too much. And he was not ready to even think about quitting for good. Then he came across harm reduction therapy and called for an initial consultation. He liked the therapist he talked with. This guy was nothing like he expected! He had a sense of humor and didn't immediately start nagging him about his use. Instead, the therapist was interested in what *he* thought. It made him realize that he wasn't really sure about anything, since he had never spent much time thinking about his life.

The one thing the therapist did do, right up front, was ask about his safety. Was he driving or riding a bike home after a long night of drinking? (Yeah.) Was he making sure that he drank water and ate food when he was doing speed? (Not much.) The therapist made it clear that his safety, and the safety of others, was important and helped him make arrangements for rides, water, and food. Other than that, nothing changed at first. He saw less of his best friend who just got married, but each time they talked the friend sounded, well, just happier somehow. He saw a TV special on how speed can damage your teeth. And he started feeling bored by his routine of bars and parties.

One night he made a list of things he'd love to do and realized that most of what showed up on the list were things that sounded very grown up: see the ruins in Mexico, learn to surf, visit Paris—all with someone there with him. No wild parties in Zanzibar with a dozen beautiful women surrounding him. He started to talk with his therapist about the things that were missing in his life. This was the beginning of the process of weighing the pros and cons of his lifestyle. After a few more sessions, he and his therapist talked about what it would feel like to stop drinking during the week. He did a decisional balance and realized that he might actually like to stop drinking after work and go to the gym with people from work instead. Once he actually signed up at the gym, he quit drinking during the week.

He also realized that he really didn't want to lose his job! He started limiting his speed use to Fridays and Saturdays, leaving Sunday to recover so he could show up to work on Monday. This was the way he tackled his patterns of alcohol and drug use: taking a look at the pros and cons of changing, then planning a series of steps to change the things that were most important to him. It didn't happen overnight, but within 6 months Tyler had quit using drugs and cut his alcohol down to cocktails with friends after work on Fridays, wine with dinner on Saturdays, and a few beers on football Sundays. He set up an online dating profile that specified that he was looking for a committed relationship. And he signed up for a surfing lesson.

Tyler didn't have a lot of emotional baggage to sort through, no particular traumas in his life, and no other serious problems that complicated his journey. He had developed a lot of habits that, over time and without his paying much attention, had gotten out of control. The only thing that he struggled with was changing his identity as the party guy. He talked a lot about how important that had been to him earlier in his life and began to see that his other friends had given up that way of being in order to have other things in their lives, things that he wanted, like a serious relationship and a variety of fun activities. And so he reluctantly moved on from his old party self—*but* he reserved the right to an occasional blowout weekend. He enjoyed those few times a year, but also enjoyed returning to the more balanced life that he had crafted.

Ruben

Ruben was struggling with both drug and health problems, all complicated by the fact that he spent a lot of time around a lot of people and yet felt lonely without a primary relationship. His history of being bullied for being gay contributed to his anxiety, which in turn was soothed by alcohol and other drugs. And his early sense of being socially rejected was being soothed by the bar and party scene. Ruben had to come to grips with some of the ghosts from his past before he could fully deal with his drug use. His therapy focused mostly on his childhood and helping him make the connections between his feeling helpless and powerless and his enjoyment of the attention he was now receiving. In addition, being rejected by his family was a source of ongoing sadness for him. He had trouble feeling good about himself when his mother and father thought that he was a "deviant." While Ruben spent a lot of time talking about these issues, we decided to reserve at least 15 minutes at the end of each session to plan for the upcoming week. He made a list of all the drugs he typically used and made as good a guess as possible about the quantities. He quickly realized that the combinations that he was using didn't necessarily work: when he used cocaine, his alcohol use went up even though he didn't particularly like the taste of most drinks. And when he used ecstasy, he became overly affectionate with men who, once the drug wore off, were not really available for anything but a quickie. And he also noticed that he was more fatigued after a weekend and worried that his HIV viral load was affected by all his use. Ruben responded very well to the non-judgmental nature of these conversations about his use. He joined with the therapist in a mutual curiosity about what, where, when, and why. He began to experiment with not using cocaine one evening and found that he drank only three beers, avoiding the sweet cocktails that he usually drank. More experiments like this led him to dramatically cut down on his use. Just paying attention to what he wanted to feel and what he ended up feeling gave him the motivation to make significant changes in a small amount of time. His health improved. He is no longer as fatigued, and he is seriously avoiding one-night stands and looking for a regular partner.

Cheryl, Tyler, and Ruben, although very different, used some of the same basic tools and strategies to get their drug use under control. Cheryl examined the reasons behind her use and spent a lot of time dealing with those underlying issues. Tyler came to grips with the fact that he was no longer living a life that he valued, and changing other habits—like joining a gym—came before the reduction in his drug use. Ruben wanted to improve his health as well as his chances of finding a partner. He started reducing both the amount and the frequency of his drug use. All three moved through the stages of change, Cheryl over a long period of time, while Tyler moved more quickly. Ruben's route was a bit more complicated, but still, within months he had made great strides.

Now Track Your Progress

On page 195 (and also online—see the end of the Contents for information on printing out additional copies) is a chart that you can use to track your progress. It corresponds to the stages of change. Note things that are big and small. We prompt you with a few examples:

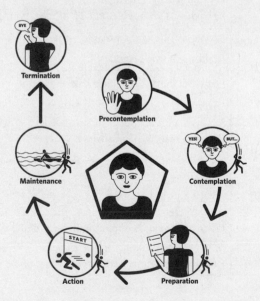

Tracking Your Progress Examples

Tasks	What You Are Accomplishing
I am listening to: (Precontemplation)	The pounding in my head when I wake up in the morning The anxiety on my kids' faces when I come home smelling like alcohol How depressed I feel after a night of Ecstasy My wife's threats to leave me My ATM withdrawals
I have learned: (Precontemplation)	My tolerance to alcohol can be reduced by a period of abstinence so I can get the same buzz with less booze. Speed constricts the capillaries in the mouth, which is why all those creepy "this is a meth head" pictures show speed users with receding gums. I would take better care of my lungs and actually waste less pot if I vaped.
I am thinking about: (Contemplation)	Why do I keep using long after I've had enough? Maybe I'd feel better if I didn't drink every day.
I have decided: (Contemplation)	I'm not going to drink hard liquor anymore. I'm going to quit smoking pot.
I am planning: (Preparation)	I've canceled a tequila-tasting party. I've told my friends that I'm cutting down on smoking pot for now. I've looked up the location of a needle exchange program. I've gotten rid of all the booze in my house. I took my dealer's number out of my cell phone. I bought a vaporizer.
I am doing: (Action)	I haven't had hard booze in 2 weeks. I went to the needle exchange.
I am taking care of myself and changing my surroundings in these ways: (Maintenance)	I've started drinking more water. I'm hanging out with an old friend who isn't into partying.
I am no longer thinking about: (Termination)	I'm not worried about gaining weight without the speed. I really like vaping so much more than smoking.

Tracking My Progress

Tasks	What You Are Accomplishing
I am listening to: (Precontemplation)	
I have learned: (Precontemplation)	
I am thinking about: (Contemplation)	
I have decided: (Contemplation)	
I am planning: (Preparation)	
I am doing: (Action)	
I am taking care of myself and changing my surroundings in these ways: (Maintenance)	
I am no longer thinking about: (Termination)	

How Do I Explain Harm Reduction to Other People?

If someone else in your life insists that you "do something" about your drug or alcohol use, you might feel you owe that person an explanation of what you are doing. Keep in mind that you don't actually have to offer quick answers—or *any* answers—until you're ready. You could say "Check in with me later" or "I'll talk to you when I've figured it out more" or the like. But if you have to answer tough questions—from parents, partners, a judge, or your boss—this short explanation will help. It can also help you organize your thoughts in conversations.

Those who care about you can read Chapter 12 or this entire book. But you might want to start by offering the summary of harm reduction here. You can simply copy pages 197–199 and hand them to people. Or you can download and print them (see the end of the Contents for information).

What's Next?

If you still aren't feeling confident in your ability to achieve the changes you'd like, the next chapter will help you find the right help. And if important others in your life need to know more than the worksheet in this chapter has provided, refer them to Chapter 12, where we speak directly to them.

Be realistic about the harm you are, and are not, doing. Don't panic, but don't underestimate. Measure your level of use with an objective eye.

Know why you use.

Know how you feel about change. Maybe you don't really want to right now.

Revisit your hierarchy of needs. Listen to your own voice about what you need and want.

Take care of things besides your drug use.

Take in positive comments from others.

Get help if you need it.

What Is Harm Reduction?

Harm reduction is a way to help people change their substance use without demanding immediate and lifelong abstinence. It uses many creative strategies to keep people alive and safe while they figure out how to develop a healthier relationship with drugs. For some people, that means abstinence; for others that means moderate or safer use.

Harm reduction takes a *health perspective,* rather than a moral or legal perspective, on drug use. Drug use is not *bad.* It is normal human behavior, and most people don't get into trouble because of it. Drug *mis*use is a habit that has gotten out of hand, or it is a signal of other co-occurring problems.

Harm reduction attends to every aspect of health—physical, mental and emotional, social, and economic. It is nonjudgmental, compassionate, and pragmatic—it starts where the person is, stays with the person through the *entire* process of change, and never *ever* kicks anyone out.

Why Do We Need Harm Reduction?

Because standard drug treatment works for only a small percentage of people who have drug problems. It is a "one-size-fits-all" system that doesn't encourage individual differences and solutions, so a lot of people get turned off. There is a need for treatment that addresses people's substance use and the issues that lie behind it. And there is desperate need for treatment that can reach people wherever they are with whatever they need *in that moment.*

Who Is Harm Reduction For?

It is for anyone who uses drugs, because *anyone* can incur harm, regardless of whether he or she has developed a serious problem.

That includes:

- People who have tried and failed at treatment attempts.

- People whose drug use is complicated by mental health or medical issues that need to be understood and treated simultaneously.

- People who want to quit but don't feel comfortable in AA or other 12-step programs.

(continued)

From *Over the Influence, Second Edition,* by Patt Denning and Jeannie Little. Copyright © 2017 The Guilford Press. Purchasers of this book can photocopy and/or download an enlarged version of this worksheet (see the box at the end of the table of contents).

- People who don't necessarily have serious drug problems but get in trouble because they don't know enough about drugs—kids going off to college, first-time users, or people who get drugs slipped into their drinks.

- People who buy drugs on the street and get contaminated drugs or drugs of uncertain composition or potency.

- People who want to understand what is causing their drug problems before deciding what the solutions are.

How Does Harm Reduction Work?

There is evidence behind all of the principles and practices of harm reduction. It works because it:

- Establishes safety—*anyone* can incur harm, regardless of whether his or her substance use rises to the level of moderate or severe *misuse.*

- Educates *everyone* about drugs and safer ways to use—knowledge without hysteria.

- Explores each person's unique relationship with drugs and understands that drug use is as complicated as the person using.

- Is realistic about change and encourages small realistic steps that can actually be achieved.

- Respects autonomy—when people have choices, they are more motivated.

- Helps people take care of themselves while they keep using—to keep them alive and healthy while they are working on change.

All of this takes place in a climate of unconditional welcome, respect, and collaboration. Self-determination is our highest value, and it leads to better health and well-being.

Dispelling Some Myths

You have to hit bottom to get serious.

People believe this because they can't understand why people don't quit despite all the evidence that they are in deep trouble. But hitting bottom is not only

(continued)

198

unnecessary—it's dangerous. Some people adapt to the bottom; others die there. The fact is, most people grow out of heavy drinking and drug use by the age of 30, usually without any help.

Abstinence is the only way.

People believe this because it's what we've been told for 50 years. And it's scary to see someone who clearly has serious problems keep on using. Quitting is safer. But abstinence isn't the only way. Many people pull themselves back to a healthier pattern. According to a large national survey on recovery from alcohol misuse, 50% of people became nonproblematic drinkers, 25% quit, and 25% continued drinking heavily.

Harm reduction is opposed to abstinence.

People believe this because harm reduction respects the individual's right to choose, including to choose drugs, and does not tell people they have to quit. Harm reduction also does not believe that people should be punished for using drugs. And harm reduction supports people who use drugs by offering them information and equipment to do so more safely.

But abstinence *is* a part of the harm reduction continuum. It is a very effective harm-reducing option, and many people end up choosing it for one or more of their drugs. It just isn't the *only* harm-reducing outcome and, in many cases, is not necessary, since so many people successfully resolve their issues with substances without quitting.

Harm reduction supports drug use and is enabling.

Harm reduction is neither for nor against drug use. Drug use is a reality. Most people in the world get intoxicated in one manner or another. Harm reduction understands drug *use* as well drug *misuse*. But that doesn't mean harm reduction *enables* people to use drugs, as if we could actually stop someone! What harm reduction enables is *safer* use. It enables informed choice. And it enables a change process that people might just stick with. That's because we love people who use drugs as much as we love anyone else. We want them to stay alive, avoid the worst harms of drug use, and have the support, the belief, and the sense of self-respect needed to make the healthiest choices possible. *In other words, harm reduction is pragmatic, and harm reduction is kind. Pragmatism and kindness promote health and change.*

11 Finding the Right Help

The opposite of addiction is not sobriety,
it's human connection.
    —JOHANN HARI, author of *Chasing the Scream:*
    The First and Last Days of the War on Drugs

Although we have encouraged you to find your own path, there are times when you need the knowledge and wisdom of others. In fact, we fully expect that this book will be only one of many resources you will use. By *resources* we mean other books, people, pets, places—things that may bring you comfort, support, encouragement, wisdom, ideas, reassurance, perspective, or hope.

In a country that values independence and self-reliance, seeking help is viewed by many people as a sign of weakness. Try not to feel embarrassed when you think about reaching out. Other people see things that we don't. Other people sometimes know more than we do, at least about *some* things. Other people might even care about us more than we care about ourselves! That's a good thing if we're neglecting or hurting ourselves. If you have any doubts about whether you need help, see the box on the facing page.

Whether you go to a program, an individual therapist or counselor, or a self-help group, the purpose of help is to provide a context in which you can develop a relationship with a professional or a group of peers with whom you can talk about your experiences, build enough trust to be truthful, and begin to address the harm in your life. The depth and duration of treatment is different for everyone. Just because your friend shares the most intimate secrets of her sex life with her therapist and you talk with yours about why your boss keeps giving you crappy assignments doesn't mean your friend is using therapy "better" than you. Just because another friend saw someone only six times and is better doesn't mean you have to rush through your therapy. And just because some people spend many years in therapy doesn't mean yours will take forever. Your therapy is as unique as your fingerprint, and it should have your fingerprints all over it!

How Do You Know
When It's Time to Seek Help?

- If your intentions to limit your use or to use more safely aren't working out, it might be time to reach out.

- If the pressure from others has become intolerable and you have to get them off your back, you might need to bring in extra resources.

- If, despite your efforts to make positive changes or at least to hold steady, your energy is waning, your skin and hair look less healthy, your hygiene is poorer rather than better, it's probably time to ask someone to check out what's going on. (A medical evaluation would be a good place to start.)

- If you are more disorganized, your mood more depressed, anxious, or up and down, your feelings angrier, sadder, or more distressed, it's probably a good time to seek out a therapist or a psychiatrist.

- If your world is crumbling around you—you're losing your job, your family, or your home, your friends are avoiding you—consider it a signal to ask a neutral outsider to help you understand where you are going wrong.

- If you are hanging around with people who take you further into harm's way—you might consider finding a place to go where you can take a break and evaluate your situation.

Right from the start, remember that help has to be *helpful,* not stressful. If the support you're being offered adds stress instead of alleviating it, look elsewhere. Help should feel good—relieving, soothing, hopeful. Even limits set by others can feel good. They provide a solid wall that you can lean on but not push over. They can keep you safe.

> Help—even when it includes limits—should feel good, like a strong wall to support you.

The first thing you should think about is whether help from others is about *you,* not them. Beware people who say, in some fashion or other, "What worked for me will work for you." No two people have the same relationship with drugs (despite popular opinion), and therefore no two people can have the same change process. Nor should others' stories of "recovery" be the yardstick by which you measure your own change process.

Also beware your own tendency to think to yourself, "Working on my problems isn't supposed to feel good! I need a program or a therapist who will be tough on me, call me on my shit, and not let me get away with anything." Most of us in this country have bought the "tough love" philoso-phy, just like we've swallowed the "pull yourself up by your bootstraps" idea. Neither is particularly effective for most people. Individual stories of "rags to riches" should not dominate your expectations of yourself.

Working with a "tough" therapist or program may be your way of accepting the anger your loved ones feel toward you. It is also possible that working with a tough therapist will be just another way to feel beaten up, in case you haven't beaten yourself up enough yet. Although it is true that reducing harm is painful, difficult, and confusing at times, your *treatment* need not be. In fact, the more painful it is, the less likely you are to stick with it. And the more enjoyable it is, the more likely you will want to go back. Therapy is supposed to reduce harm, not re-create it for $100

> Find a program or therapist that is not dogmatic and not single-mindedly attached to abstinence as the only way to resolve problems with drugs.

an hour. The most important thing is to find a program or therapist that is not dogmatic about a single model or single-mindedly attached to abstinence as the only way to resolve problems with drugs.

How to Decide What Help You Need

First of All, Who Decides?

Hopefully, you do! Many people know what they want and need and, given free rein to be honest and choose their own goals, they will choose the best course of action. And people should be ready **to hear your decisions**. The literature on goal choice shows that the more people choose their own goals, the more successful they are. But if you don't have a clear sense of direction, or if you aren't confident in the progress you've made so far, this is the time for outside help.

What Goes into a Decision to Seek Formal Treatment?

The question is not just "What do I need?" It is also "What will be help-ful and not harmful?" Most important is to find a place where you will be accepted as you are right now.

If a professional is evaluating you for treatment, recommendations will be made based on your level of use and the severity of your problems. In general, the greater the severity (amount and dangerousness) of your sub-stance use, the more critical the medical or psychiatric complications, and the weaker the "recovery" environment, the higher the intensity of treatment (hospital detox or 28-day rehab, for example) recommended.

This is all very well, but your *motivation and readiness* to change and *what you want* should always be the primary consideration, except in cases when safety requires immediate attention. *In other words, self-determination should always be honored.* When people are not ready to change, they are more likely to "vote with their feet" and leave a program, no matter

> Motivation should always be the primary consideration in treatment recommendations.

how severe their problems. This means that high-intensity placements for those who aren't motivated might be wasted.

The Importance of Options

If you are to be the decision maker about what kind of help you get, it is critical that you have options. Choice is empowering, and it leads to better outcomes. *Even if you are mandated to treatment by a boss, a judge, or a family*

> Choice is empowering, and it leads to better outcomes.

intervention, you need options. In the rest of this chapter we give you tips on how to choose treatment and what questions to ask when you apply.

Three Essential Considerations

In harm reduction, we make determinations or recommendations based on three important considerations—safety, structure, and direction. You can evaluate any treatment program, group, or counselor in light of these three considerations.

Safety

Safety is our first concern, as we have said many times, and any program you choose should prioritize your safety over and above other changes you make. Syringe exchange programs, safe injection facilities, naloxone distribution and overdose prevention training, accurate drug and safe use information, and substance use management and moderation coaching are the foundations of harm reduction. Any program, regardless of its stance on abstinence as a goal of treatment, should include information on all of these life-saving options. Even if your own goal is abstinence, you might return to using at times and need access to information and services for active users.

Structure

When people refer to "structure" in substance use treatment, often what they mean is putting someone in a *restrictive* environment that will eliminate risk, regulate behavior, and prevent any contact with psychoactive substances. That is, they will ensure abstinence by restricting participants' access to the outside world, often including restricting the use of phones or computers. The extent of restrictiveness in a program is often what is meant by the level of *intensity* of treatment.

Direction

Directive programs or therapists tell people what to do and how to do it. The vast majority of programs (rehabs, outpatient treatment, and self-help groups) prescribe a lifetime of abstinence from psychoactive drugs. Most also prescribe a lifetime of membership in a 12-step group, a sponsor, and working the steps. Standard treatment also tends to be directive, with the same groups and activities required for all participants, including time lines or stages that people move through based on behavior and program adherence. Often this direction comes with exhortations that failure to follow "the program" will lead to "jails, institutions and death." This dire prediction comes from the *NA White Booklet* put out by Narcotics Anonymous in 1976.

Although harm reduction values self-determination above all else, we do understand that, at some times, people need high levels of structure and direction. It can be a relief to be kept out of harm's way. But many people who are reading this book have tried and failed with such programs. Here are some questions to ask if you are seeking a high-intensity program:

- To what extent does the program exert control over participants' activities?

- Does it restrict contact with the "outside world" and activities within the program?

- Are people free to come and go as they please?

- To what extent does it tell participants what to do?

- Does it prescribe the goals *and* direct the methods to achieve those goals? Support the clients' choices (short of harm to self and others) and methods?

- To what extent are punitive sanctions imposed for failure to "comply" with program rules and expectations?

- Does the program punish, humiliate, or dismiss? Or does it applaud the strength displayed by someone who resists?

- What about harm reduction? Does the program educate its participants about safe drug use tactics?

The Challenge Is Balance

The challenge for any treatment program is to provide the right amount of structure and direction to guide each person's change process without violating the person's right to self-determination, thwarting the need for autonomy, or robbing the participant of the right to get treatment that has the best chance of working. Each person needs a different level of safety, structure, and direction, and the need for each will change over time. The key is to find a program that is flexible enough to adapt along with each individual as he or she changes. As a general rule, regardless of the program, we recommend the following ground rules:

- The structure should be consensual, not coerced.

- No program should ever be punitive or shaming.

- The level of structure should be based on either your therapeutic needs or your safety.

What Are the Treatment Options?

Despite the public perception that rehab is the place to go when your drug use gets out of hand, the generally accepted professional wisdom is that people should try the least restrictive environment first (unless serious safety concerns or a mandate interferes). If your changes are too dramatic or come too quickly, you might not be able to integrate them into your real life. There is a rebound effect—people tend to bounce in and out of "rehab" several times—which is an exercise in failure and disappointment. There are two main decisions to be made: the *level of intensity* that you need or want and the *type* of treatment that you prefer.

Level of Intensity

Restrictive programs offer a level of containment that can promote safety for people who are impulsive and whose substance use is potentially dangerous to self or others. Restriction (and direction, described below) can be desirable for people who desperately want to break habits or for people who need medical intervention and monitoring. It is also appealing to families who just want their loved one's behavior to stop, to bring order to chaos. Just as a child who is about to run out in the street needs to be picked up and put indoors, adults sometimes need to be gotten out of harm's way. And, for people who can retain the image of the Breathalyzer, the urine sample bottle, or the ankle bracelet, these "big brother" devices can be effective deterrents against unwanted behavior. Containment can provide reassurance that is emotionally calming. Being kept out of harm's way can make it easier to think and plan your future.

On the other hand, being restricted can retraumatize people whose lives have been arbitrarily controlled by others; who have been abused as children or as adults; who have been institutionalized; who have been terrorized in their families, neighborhoods, or countries; or who have been locked up in jails and prisons. Since most people who persistently misuse substances have trauma in their histories, *anyone* might have sensitivities that would render restrictive programs more harmful than helpful. (In the box on the facing page, we offer a guide to the different levels of treatment.)

Any program can be directive, regardless of its restrictiveness, although there is more chance of it in a restrictive residential environment. Even medium-intensity programs might, to varying degrees, use monitoring devices, thus extending their reach beyond the physical bounds of the program. If participation is coerced, regardless of the intensity of the program, the whole process is involuntary.

Types of Treatment

We divide the treatment options into three categories—*disease model, cognitive-behavioral,* and *harm reduction* programs, followed by a section on *self-help groups,* which can fall under any of the three models. Within each section programs can range along the continuum of structure from very to not at all restrictive and directive, with harm reduction programs and self-help groups sitting on the less restrictive end of the continuum. They are all represented in both residential and outpatient settings, although harm reduction is rarely practiced in residential treatment because state laws forbid drug use and drinking in licensed facilities. The major differences are whether programs insist on abstinence as the goal of treatment, whether they use faith-based or evidence-based practices, and whether they help people identify and embrace the full range of harm-reducing goals. In the box on pages 208–209

Levels of Treatment

- *High intensity*: residential (hospitals and other medical detoxification programs, usually short-term); "rehab," usually 28 days, but sometimes longer; or intensive outpatient (sometimes called partial hospitalization)—5 days a week, several hours a day.

- *Medium Intensity*: intensive outpatient that is 9 hours a week, usually groups and one counseling session 3 days a week; regular outpatient programs that might consist of one group a week and one or no individual counseling sessions.

- *Low intensity*: self-help groups, which fall along a continuum from abstinence based to harm reduction based (see page 215 for a list of self-help options); other self-help resources, including books, manuals, and websites (see the list of recommended readings and websites in the Resources at the back of the book); sober living houses where you go out to work or other daily activities.

Medication-Assisted Treatment

Medication-assisted treatment (MAT) refers to addiction medicine—the prescribing of medicines that replace or help to reduce cravings for drugs that you are having problems with (see Chapter 8). MAT can be included in any of the programs listed above or can occur alongside them.

we discuss the effectiveness of the various options and offer some warnings about rehab programs.

Disease-Model Programs

Often we call disease-model programs "traditional treatment," because the disease model is the dominant model of addiction and treatment in the United States. It has been blended with the 12 steps of Alcoholics Anonymous: 77% of all substance use treatment programs are based on the 12 steps. Bear in mind that the 12 steps are *faith based,* so most treatment in the United States is therefore faith-based treatment. Here are some things you should expect from disease-model programs:

- *Insistence that abstinence from all substances is the only way to "recover" from drug and alcohol problems*: Given that the characteristics of "addiction," according to the disease model, are denial and loss of control (or a hijacked brain),

How Effective Is Disease-Model Drug Treatment?

Outcomes of drug treatment have always been measured in terms of abstinence rates. They are not impressive. They usually hover around 25%, according to estimates. The only scientifically designed survey of drug treatment in the United States, conducted by the federal Substance Abuse and Mental Health Services Administration (SAMHSA) and completed in 1998, found abstinence rates of 21% several years after the completion of treatment. It is much more difficult to find out how many people *never complete* the treatment programs they enter, but it is the majority. The same study, interestingly, found much more impressive results when it measured *harm reduction* outcomes. These included *reduction* in drug use, criminal activity, unemployment, loss of children to the child welfare system, medical crises, and other quality-of-life issues. Improvement rates ranged from 23 to 43% in these areas. We can only imagine how much better treatment attendance and reduction in various harms would be if people got to *pick* their goals. Research in Europe, where there are real alternatives between abstinence and controlled use, indicate positive results. Furthermore, most people, given a choice, decide to work toward abstinence!

Traditional drug treatment programs also tend to undertreat other problems, such as depression and anxiety. Some think that if you get too comfortable, you won't remember why you're there and you'll relapse. The rule of thumb is: no therapy until you have been in "recovery" for a year. Some programs disapprove of the use of prescribed psychiatric medications, and many don't allow you to be on methadone (or other addiction medicines) either, despite the fact that using medicines specifically for your substance issues could be very helpful to your efforts to stop or reduce your use.

It has been found to be unconstitutional to mandate attendance at 12-step meetings. Because of the obvious religious components, several courts of appeal have stated that such a requirement violates our constitutional right to the separation of church and state and religious freedom.

Three Cautions

Rehab: The "Miracle" of 28 Days

There is no rational reason why a typical rehab program lasts for 28 days. This magic number has been derived from changing insurance requirements. Long ago, inpatient and residential rehabilitation programs lasted for months or years, but as the insurance industry got involved, the decision was to fund for only "detoxification and stabilization," not ongoing treatment! Unfortunately, this 28-day stay has been sold to us as the perfect program: we will come out changed forever! Needless to say, most of us can't make lasting changes in complex behaviors in so little time. And we have read countless stories of celebrities cycling in and out of expensive rehabs. Their stories are not unique.

Treatment Trauma

Over the years we have worked with hundreds of people who have tried (or been mandated to attend) traditional programs. Some of these people report experiences that made them feel so ashamed, hopeless, or lazy that they are actually suffering from being in the program! Others haven't been allowed to take medications for their psychiatric symptoms and have suffered years of depression or anxiety while they try to fix their "character defects." We now use the term *treatment trauma* to refer to the feelings of guilt and shame, or anger, that so many people report to us. We spend considerable amounts of therapeutic time helping people undo some of the negative self-concepts and feelings of failure so they can gain enough self-confidence to try again.

A Special Caution about Teen Rehabs, Wilderness Programs, and Therapeutic Boarding Schools

There has been a growing industry of programs for troubled teens. Some of them are undoubtedly helpful, but a large percentage are harmful to the point of being abusive and in some cases lethal. Many have been forcibly closed down by licensing boards because of infractions ranging from physical abuse to isolation and intimidation. If you are a parent seeking treatment for a child, take a close look at any program, including an onsite visit, before committing.

Four authors who have studied the substance use treatment industry exhaustively are Stanton Peele, Maia Szalavitz, Anne Fletcher, and Lance Dodes. They all have excellent books in which they discuss their experience or their study of treatments and their effectiveness. Their books are listed in the Resources at the back of the book.

there is simply no room for moderate or controlled use and certainly not for acceptance of safer drug use as an acceptable goal.

- *Zero tolerance for drug use or relapse while in the program*: In most places, any drug use during the program will get you kicked out.

- *Confrontation of "denial"*: Unfortunately, accusing people of "denial" and forcefully pointing out the harms of their use is often the technique of choice. You might not be able to tell how strenuous this confrontational approach will be from a phone conversation. Some treatment programs, especially some of the older "therapeutic communities," use confrontation, punishment, and humiliation to break down and transform your "addictive personality" (there's no such thing, by the way). This is the ultimate in tough love. Since we believe that most drug users have already been traumatized, stigmatized, and shamed, we find the idea of breaking someone's spirit in this way to be horrifying. Certain people do benefit from such an extreme approach: they overcome serious addictions and even criminal behavior patterns. By now you know that this is not an approach we endorse, especially for people who have been oppressed or traumatized.

• *Mandated 12-step participation*: All 12-step–based programs want you to become part of the AA or NA community ("the fellowship"). When we wrote the original edition of this book, 93% of programs were based on the 12 steps; now it is 77%, as noted above. When you're in one of these programs, you are required to attend 12-step meetings as a condition of your participation. If you are going to use traditional treatment and/or self-help programs, you must either decide that you believe what they are saying and entrust yourself to the program, the counselors, and the other participants or find other skeptics like yourself who can help you deal with the conflicts that will arise. A good therapist should be able to help you manage these conflicts. Programs are increasingly allowing clients to participate in other, non–12-step peer groups like SMART Recovery and LifeRing.

Cognitive-Behavioral Programs

Cognitive-behavioral treatment takes the perspective that conditioned responses, thoughts, and/or beliefs are the main determinants of behavior. A conditioned response is an automatic response to a familiar stimulus. The most famous example is Pavlov's dog, who learned to salivate whenever he heard the food bell regardless of whether the food was there. This is what people mean when they talk about "cues" or "triggers." The food bell is a *cue* that food is coming. After a while, the dog associates the bell with the food and salivates whenever he hears the bell. This then becomes a habit or a pattern—an automatic behavior that the dog (or you) no longer thinks about. The same is true if you see an advertisement for a particular beer that you like. You might find yourself craving that beer (having thoughts and desires that are essentially the same as salivating). Cognitive therapists added the idea that thoughts and beliefs maintain habits and that what is learned can be unlearned if you help people become conscious of the association between their thoughts and their behaviors.

Many cognitive-behavioral treatments are evidence based. They have either been developed out of research or evolved in practice and then been formally studied. Some have been turned into manuals. You might be familiar with the many helpful manuals written for the general public—those that focus on managing stress or anger, building healthy relationships, or maintaining healthy diet and exercise patterns. These manuals are very similar to what practitioners of cognitive-behavioral treatments might use, and often there are workbooks for clients.

> Cognitive-behavioral treatments are often evidence-based treatments.

Some of the better-known cognitive-behavioral models that we respect and/or use ourselves include:

- The *stages of change* model is well explained in previous chapters. Many programs are familiar with the stages of change, and some use it in their treatment. The challenge is with programs that presuppose abstinence as the only goal of treatment. They must get comfortable working with active substance users and comfortable talking about the cons *and* the pros of drug use. A good self-help book by the developers of the stages of change model is *Changing for Good* (see the Resources).

- *Seeking Safety* is a counseling model that was developed for people who misuse substances and have histories of trauma. It has historically been abstinence focused, but more recently its developer, Lisa Najavits, has embraced harm reduction by recognizing that people will not just quit because someone thinks they should and that substances serve as an important coping mechanism for many people. She has published a book for the general public on this method (you can find it in the Resources section).

- *Dialectical behavior therapy (DBT)* is a very helpful treatment for people with difficulty managing strong emotions, many of whom have suffered traumatic events. Over the last few years it has also been applied to people with substance use problems.

- *Motivational interviewing* evolved as a client-centered and supportive counseling approach to help people resolve ambivalence and develop motivation to change.

- For families, *Community Reinforcement and Family Training (CRAFT)* is a method for helping families to help their loved ones, based on science and compassion.

Most cognitive-behavioral programs focus on the goal of abstinence, but the good ones understand and embrace three fundamental things: the gradual nature of change, the predominance of co-occurring disorders, and the value of the therapeutic relationship. They do not kick people out for engaging in the very behavior that brought them to treatment, they simultaneously treat substance misuse and emotional or psychological problems, and they work very hard to maintain a connection even if the client is trying very hard to leave the program. While often useful, we find them limited by the lack of attention paid to the very real medical benefits of substance use, its unconscious meanings, and the attachment that people have to it.

Harm Reduction Programs

Harm reduction therapy is the treatment model of the harm reduction movement. It is the treatment model described in this book, so you are pretty familiar with it by now. It integrates cognitive-behavioral strategies in the context of exploring the self-medicating properties of drugs, the meaning of each person's relationship with drugs, and the context in which each person lives. A comprehensive list of harm reduction programs is in the Resources section, but for example, harm reduction programs include:

- Needle exchange programs
- Safe injection facilities (SIFs)
- Drug education programs in schools that offer real, not "Just Say No" drug information
- Harm reduction therapists
- Any program that helps clients select from a wide range of nonabstinence goals

Harm reduction programs fall on the least restrictive and directive end of the continuum, with participants choosing not only their goals but also the pace and the intensity of their participation. We refer to this as "dosing"—just as people dose themselves with drugs as they wish, they also dose themselves with treatment, coming and going as they see fit with no penalty. As we hope you have gathered from this book, harm reduction is *multidirectional*—safety, moderation, abstinence, and/or attending to issues other than substance use are all worthy directions for change. It is client directed and empowering. Because self-determination is a core value of harm reduction, we see our role as facilitators rather than directors of a person's change process. We make recommendations only after considering the strength of the therapeutic alliance *and only after being invited by the client.*

It seems somewhat redundant to discuss what to expect from harm reduction programs, since this entire book is a *virtual* harm reduction program, but we want to highlight features that we think most distinguish harm reduction from other programs:

• **Focus on health and safety, regardless of your desire to change anything else:** Switching to clean needles—"one needle, one shot"—is truly good enough. So is not driving under the influence. As is waiting to get high until after the kids go to bed. We stress basics like eating, drinking water, and getting enough sleep alongside using drugs. If you or someone else wants more than that, that's fine, or even important, but a *harm reduction* program will not impose expectations on you about what might be best.

• **Client centered, client specific, and client directed:** You create your own program in collaboration with your therapist or counselor. Together you address issues in the order that you consider most important.

• **Trauma informed:** We recognize that many of our clients will have had traumatic experiences that must be attended to. This includes making sure that administrative policies as well as clinical practices do no harm and help the client reduce the symptoms of traumatic experiences.

• **Integrated treatment of co-occurring problems:** Because there is growing pressure to treat people who have "dual diagnoses," however, it is possible that any program you call might allow use of psychiatric medications and might even have a physician available to prescribe them. Harm reduction programs also offer medication-assisted treatment (MAT), or work closely with programs that do. MAT refers to the use of medications to treat substance misuse, typically to either replace your substance of choice or reduce cravings. Medications are especially useful with physiological dependence or chaotic use. These medicines are discussed in Chapter 8.

• **Substance use management:** Use of a variety of options for change, including safer use, controlled use, moderation, abstinence, or a combination, with different options for different drugs. (We discuss substance use management in great detail in Chapter 8.)

> Harm reduction treatment is integrative, client directed, and offers a wide menu of options for change.

Self-Help Groups

Self-help, more properly called *mutual aid,* groups are many and varied. These groups are all about mutual support by and for people who have problems in common. By definition, mutual aid groups are not professionally led. In the case of alcohol and other drug problems, they are supportive groups of peers who come together to help one another manage their problems with substances. Alcoholics Anonymous and its sister programs are, by far, the most widespread of all these groups. A number of other programs that offer alternatives to the spiritual approach of AA have sprung up in recent decades. Most expect their members to have abstinence as their goal, although most do not reject people who have not achieved it.

> "Self-help" doesn't mean you're on your own. It just means these groups are facilitated by peers, not professionals. They are more properly called *mutual aid* groups.

These groups fall on their own continuum of restrictiveness and direction. They also range from disease model to cognitive-behavioral to harm reduction based. While they are not physically restrictive, attendance is sometimes mandated. *Reporting*—for example, by the show of hands for people who are "newcomers" at 12-step meetings or by the sharing of the number of drinks and drinking days one has had in the last week at Moderation Management meetings—is an accountability device that, if internalized and remembered while away from the group, provides a sense that the group is always present. In 12-step groups, goals *and* methods are clearly prescribed. Both Moderation Management and SMART Recovery (Self-Management and Recovery Training) have a clear *direction* or *prescribed goal*—moderation of alcohol use or abstinence, respectively—but the structure of meetings is not directive. They function as facilitated discussions where people can explore their relationship with substances, evaluate their individual risk situations, and set their own goals. The HAMS (Harm Reduction, Abstinence, and Moderation Support) network is harm reduction's mutual support group for alcohol. It encourages people to choose safety, moderation, *or* abstinence, and to define moderate drinking for themselves.

How to Look for Treatment

As we said earlier in this chapter, we recommend that you try the least restrictive program first. Staying close to home and continuing with your

Support/Mutual Aid Group Options

Harm Reduction Support

- Community-based groups (facilitated by staff or volunteers at many harm reduction organizations)

- *Over the Influence* book clubs (also hosted by organizations)

- HAMS (Harm Reduction, Abstinence, and Moderation Support) holds online meetings and is specific to alcohol, though people discuss other drugs too (*www.hamsnetwork.org*).

Moderation Support

- Moderation Management holds in-person and online meetings. It is a program specifically for alcohol moderation (*www.moderation.org*).

Abstinence Support

- SMART (Self-Management and Recovery Treatment), in person and online. SMART is part of the harm reduction continuum of options because, although it is an abstinence-oriented program, it supports self-selected goals.

- Women for Sobriety holds groups and forums in person and online. It, too, is a secular organization (*www.womenforsobriety.org*).

- LifeRing Secular Recovery: LifeRing refers to itself as sober, secular, and self-directed (*www.lifering.org*).

- Secular Organization for Sobriety is a nonreligious alternative that is located in many parts of the country (*www.sossobriety.org*).

- Refuge Recovery is "a mindfulness-based addiction recovery community." It has meetings in most states (*www.refugerecovery.org*).

> Changes that are integrated into your life will feel most natural and will be most sustainable.

regular activities at the same time you get help to change your relationship with drugs will help you integrate changes into your life immediately. Changes that are integrated into your life will feel most natural and will be most sustainable.

Questions to Ask to Make Sure You Get What You Need

Even a few well-chosen questions will give you a feel for what the program is like and whether you might be able to benefit from it, or at least tolerate it and learn a little.

1. What is the philosophy of your program? (disease model, cognitive-behavioral, harm reduction?)

2. Do you require attendance at 12-step meetings?

3. Are you an abstinence-only program or do you help people with harm reduction goals, including moderation?

4. Do you drug test?

5. What activities do you have in the program?

6. Can I opt out of certain activities?

7. How many groups do you have compared to individual counseling sessions?

8. Are your staff licensed professionals? Do you offer a psychiatric consultation and prescribe psychiatric medications? Do you offer medication-assisted treatment?

9. Can I stay on the medications my outside doctor prescribes, including benzodiazepines for anxiety?

10. Do you have specialized services to treat trauma, depression, bipolar disorder, and so forth?

11. Will you work with my therapist and doctor while I am here?

12. How much contact can I have with my family and friends?

13. What happens if I use while in the program?

Training Your Therapist

Many programs and therapists do not identify as harm reduction practitioners. Nevertheless, many practice harm reduction by treating substance use issues alongside any other issues of concern. In other words, they do not segregate your problems, and they seek to understand the meaning and the role of drugs in your life. Many therapists are willing to read something that you suggest so that they can understand harm reduction. Show them this book. Talk about it with them. Give them the professional reading list from the Resources. We have also written a very readable book for professionals on this topic: *Practicing Harm Reduction Psychotherapy* (Guilford Press, 2012).

What's Next?

The next, and final, chapter is written to your family and friends. In it, we help you start the process of teaching them about harm reduction. We talk to them about moving away from "tough love" and instead basing their decisions on what they need, what they can manage, and what they value most. We suggest the possibility that they can love you *and* set limits. And that those limits don't need to be tough; they just need to be authentic and consistent. If you want, you can share it with the people in your life who don't understand drug use and don't understand harm reduction. Or you can keep it to yourself. It's your choice.

Help has to be helpful, and it has to be about you.

Structure and limits can be like a strong wall to lean against; they should never be punitive.

You get to ask a program or a therapist all the questions you want—*you* are the client. It's your treatment, and it's your future!

12 A Letter to Family and Friends of People Who Use Drugs

There are the facts, then there's the truth.
And your facts are never going to change my truth.
—REV. EDWIN SANDERS, Metropolitan
Interdenominational Church,
Nashville, Tennessee, First Response
Center and Partners for Life

Loving someone who has an alcohol or other drug problem can be excruciating. If you just found out about a loved one's problems with alcohol or drugs, you may be frightened. If you've been dealing with a drug-using loved one for a long time, and nothing you do or say seems to make a difference, you weather profound helplessness, frustration, or anger. You end up struggling with questions about loyalty, love, support, and limits. What you want is solutions. Right now. And what you've been told—to set limits and practice tough love—may or may not feel like the answer.

I (Patt) have been a therapist for 40 years. I wasn't trained specifically to work with drug problems. I developed this specialty when I worked with hundreds of young men with AIDS in the first HIV clinic in the country. Years later, after starting the Center for Harm Reduction Therapy in 2000 with Jeannie, I began getting calls from concerned friends and family members who had tried Al Anon and other self-help groups and needed something more. I realized that we were offering state-of-the-art alternative treatment for drug users, and I wanted to be able to offer the same kind of help to those who love them.

I have consulted with dozens of families and friendship networks over the past 10 years. The stories I have heard convinced me that a family member's experience with a drug-using loved one is just as complicated as the user's relationship with his or her drugs. The assistance that I have been able to offer comes from what I have learned through many conversations about what isn't working and what families and friends need.

The advice you have been given by support groups, friends, and acquaintances who care about you is informed by the dominant cultural view of drugs and drug use:

- Don't enable them—they need "tough love."
- Don't protect them—they need to "hit bottom" before they'll get it.
- Don't trust them—"all addicts lie."

If you do any of these things, you are codependent. You are suffering from the same disease they are.

But "having a problem should not be equated with being the problem," say Judith Gordon and Kimberly Barrett in their powerful critique of the "codependency movement." And *you're* thinking, "But that's my son, my mother, my grandfather, the big brother who had my back, my cousins who I spent every minute with when I was a kid, my life partner! I can't turn my back on them." You also understand the suffering behind the person's drug use—whether it is mental illness, loss and grief, low self-esteem, terror of not being able to take care of him- or herself, or myriad other vulnerabilities. If only you could take the pain away, he or she wouldn't need drugs anymore.

You very well might be right. And your feelings of love, compassion, and loyalty are good. They are the feelings of people who are humane and who believe that part of being human is to take care of others. Including sometimes putting the needs of others before yours. Self-sacrifice is one of the core values of religions, heroes, and mothers the world over. It is revered, not despised. Except when it comes to the sacrifices you make to care for a loved one who uses and misuses drugs.

There are several problems with the standard advice. Tough love is neither (and it feels horrible to everyone). Tough love is often a reaction to years of anger at yourself for having endured for so long. It can feel more like a punishment than a strategy. Hitting bottom *is not* motivating—it's dangerous and demoralizing. People suffer horrific consequences and sometimes die at the bottom. Interventions backfire—it can take years for a family to recover from the rupture caused by an intervention. And while the treatment a person is forced into might work, there are other ways to get there that cause less harm.

You have also been told: They're addicts or alcoholics. They have to quit all drugs for the rest of their lives, with the help of AA or NA. If they don't, inevitably they will face "jails, institutions, or death." And finally, if they don't listen to these instructions, you have to conduct the aforementioned intervention.

But These Things Just Don't Work—Why Not?

Most people do not go to treatment, and almost half of them say it's because they aren't ready to quit. Of those who do, more than half drop out. And for people who try 12-step meetings, the dropout rate is 90%. The problem is, most programs have only one story, and, despite popular and official opinion, that story does not fit most people. There is no room for the possibility that drugs are a *solution* to other, bigger, problems. Most people who misuse drugs have something else going on. How many times have you told doctors and treatment professionals things like "I don't think it's just his addiction. I know there's something else serious going on." "He was an isolated child." "Her father disappeared for long periods of time." "He's been having rages since he got back from Iraq." "She hasn't been the same since her husband died."

For treatment to be effective, it has to be flexible enough to work with each individual's relationship with drugs and to address *all* of the issues facing a person. When it doesn't, people *resist,* which is their way of saying "This doesn't work for *me;* you don't *get* me. I do have ideas of what's wrong, and I have to figure it out in my own time."

What Can You Do?

You can practice harm reduction. Harm reduction is about damage control. It is about keeping people alive while they find their way. It invites individuals to tell their story in their own way. It respects self-determination and offers a collaboration to find solutions together. And it is realistic about how long it takes to change. Harm reduction is about motivation, not coercion. It recognizes that the idea of powerlessness doesn't appeal to most people; rather, feeling powerful is essential to lasting change. For all of these reasons, harm reduction can engage any and every drug user in a process of self-understanding and change.

Harm reduction suggests that you undertake the same kind of balanced evaluation of your needs and your options for taking care of yourself that we offer to drug users. We suggest that you weigh the pros and cons of your options so that whatever action you take reflects the complexity of your relationship with your son, daughter, partner, parent, cousin, best friend, or colleague. Just as the drug user needs to respect the complexity of his or her relationship with drugs before making decisions that will actually *work,* you need to respect the complexity of your relationship with the drug user.

Harm reduction does not believe that you have to end a relationship to improve it. Nor is "abstinence" necessarily seen as the basis for an improved life. An "addict" does not have to "hit bottom" to become motivated to make positive changes, and nor do you. Harm reduction is a *both/and* approach. You can love your child *and* kick her out of the house. You can kick her out of the house *and* pay her rent somewhere else. In these ways you can continue to love and support her and limit the damage she can do to your marriage, your house, and your other kids. In other words, you can make changes in your relationship with your loved one way before you are completely worn out. In fact you should.

Harm Reduction Principles for Family and Friends

Promises only cause problems: The cycle of hope and despair is perpetuated by demanding promises to change that are repeatedly not met.

There are no rules except the ones you make: You get to decide how to love. If paying a person's rent to prevent him being homeless *and* drug dependent helps you sleep at night, do it!

You cannot enable drug use (unless you are supplying them): You can only enable love, support, and survival.

Base your actions on your values: Loyalty, understanding, compassion, generosity, and humility ("There but for the grace of God go I") are the values of altruism and heroism. If these are your values, honor them.

Base your actions on what you can manage: Small changes in yourself can lead to larger steps.

You have triggers too: You've been traumatized and will overreact at times.

Any limits you set are about *you*: Set limits based on what *you* need, not what you think will make *them* change! You will be more authentic and, ultimately, more successful.

I hope that this brief message will help you make a harm reduction plan for yourself. All of the principles and techniques in this book can be used as a guide for you, a guide that can lead to changes you may not be totally satisfied with, but that you know represent the best you can do. I hope that this letter, and this book, will enable you to return to a life that is less fraught and more powerful and optimistic.

Patt Denning

What You Should Know about Drugs

A Quick Reference

We neither condemn nor condone the use of any particular drug. We simply recognize that people use them and always have, whether we think they should or not. We want people to stay alive, to be as safe as possible, to enjoy their lives, and to have relationships with people who are interested in their well-being. It is with these values in mind that we have taken as much care as possible with the following compendium.

Some of the sources listed in the Resources give conflicting information. In some cases, research is poor because most of the drugs are illegal. In other cases, the drugs are too new to allow long-term observation of how they work. We have done our best to select reputable sources, but as in all things, we cannot guarantee that we have found the best sources or that your individual experience will match what we say here. We will highlight the ones we rely on most often. Consulting a physician or pharmacist is a good idea if you're uncertain, but for many reasons, it is also a good idea for people to do their own research. Just Say Know!

General Concepts and Terminology

What Is a Drug?

To quote Andrew Weil, who has been studying drugs and health for decades, a drug is "any substance that in small amounts produces significant changes in the body, mind, or both." A *psychoactive* drug is one that crosses the blood–brain barrier to cause alterations in mood, perception, or brain function. The blood–brain barrier can be crossed only by drugs that are soluble in fat (aspirin, for example, is not and is therefore not psychoactive). Psychoactive drugs range from prescribed medications, alcohol, and stimulants such as methamphetamine to common solvents such as paint thinner or glue.

Drugs come in many different forms. To put it simply, some are *natural,* like coca leaves, coffee beans and tea leaves, cannabis (marijuana), tobacco, opium, and khat. Others are *extracted* or processed from their original natural forms, such as cocaine from coca leaves, beer from barley and malt, whiskey from corn or rye, and codeine from opium. Still others are *synthetic,* meaning that they have been made of molecules and chemical combinations that aren't found in nature. LSD, MDMA (ecstasy), ketamine, Dilaudid, and methamphetamine are examples of synthetic drugs.

What Is the Difference between a Drug and a Food?

Sometimes very little. We commonly think of tea, coffee, and chocolate as part of our diet, but in fact they contain the world's most-consumed psychoactive substance—caffeine. Sugar is a food, but it is notorious for causing changes in activity level and mood. Some historians suggest that our ancient use of mind-altering substances may have been, in part, as a source of nutrients—to ward off hunger or fatigue or to replenish neurotransmitters (brain chemicals) in situations where food was scarce or didn't travel or keep well.

> *Important Questions for Drug Users to Ask*
> - "What is it? What does it do?"
> - "Is it legal or illegal? What are the penalties for possess or selling it?"
> - "How can I use it? What are the risks and benefits from different methods of use?"
> - "How fast does it take effect? When does it usually reach its peak effect? How long does the effect last?"
> - "How long will its presence be detectable in my body?"
> - "What happens when alcohol, medications, or other drugs are combined with it?"
> - "What can I do to maximize my enjoyment while minimizing the potential negatives?"

Dependence, Tolerance, and Withdrawal

Tolerance refers to the process of physiological adaptation, whereby the body and brain attempt to establish homeostasis (balance) in the presence of a new chemical. The brain adapts by producing chemical changes and by learning to behave under altered circumstances. Tolerance has developed when consuming the same amount of a drug produces a lessened effect, so that to get the same effect as before, one must consume larger amounts of the drug. Tolerance can develop to some effects and not to others; for example, a person can become tolerant to the sedative, sleep-inducing effects of Valium but not usually to its anxiety-reducing effects.

Cross-tolerance happens when tolerance develops to all drugs in the same class (for example, alcohol and benzodiazepines both work, in part, on the GABA system; they have similar sedating effects, and benzodiazepines can be used to help someone go through alcohol detoxification).

Dependence means *physiological dependence,* which is characterized only by tolerance and/or withdrawal and may have nothing to do with psychological dependence (which people usually call addiction). For example, if you take pain medicine over a long period of time, you will eventually become physically dependent on it and will have to stop slowly to avoid suffering withdrawal. The same is true of some antidepressant medications, such as Paxil. However, you are better off taking it than not. In other words, if a medicine makes you function better, you are not *addicted* to it, even if your body becomes physically dependent on it.

Withdrawal refers to physical or psychological symptoms that appear when the drug is discontinued. Usually these symptoms are opposite of the drug's effects. For example, opioids cause constipation, and diarrhea is a symptom of opioid withdrawal. Long-term or heavy use of alcohol and benzodiazepines raises the seizure threshold in the brain by causing neurons to fire more rapidly to maintain balance (homeostasis) in the presence of the depressant effects of the substances; during withdrawal, the risk of seizure is increased during the lapse of time before neurons slow down again.

Substance Use Disorders

The older way of talking about problems with alcohol and other drugs are terms such as *abuse, dependence,* and *addiction.* The current view (described in DSM-5) is both more precise and more informative. One has a substance use disorder when the use of a drug for *nonmedical* purposes results in health or social problems and/or continued use despite negative consequences. Substance use disorders can be mild, moderate, or severe. We use the term *substance misuse* to cover the full range of patterns, most of which do *not* reach the threshold of a substance use disorder. For example, you can misuse alcohol by drinking too much occasionally, but if you haven't had any negative consequences (other than a hangover and some regrets), you don't qualify as having a diagnosable substance use disorder.

Gateway Drugs

This is more myth than fact. A gateway drug is one you use earlier in life that supposedly puts you at risk for using "harder" drugs later. A big focus of the gateway drug theory is marijuana. But research over the past 20 years has proven that marijuana use does not lead to the use of other drugs. The vast majority of people who have used marijuana have never used a "harder" drug. According to the National Academy of Sciences, there is "no conclusive evidence that the drug effects of marijuana are causally linked to the subsequent abuse of other drugs." While the rates of use of marijuana have increased steadily over the past 20 years, use of other illicit drugs has declined. (Marijuana may be more accurately described as an "exit drug"—people use it to get off alcohol, heroin, and other substances, or to at least decrease their use of those drugs.) Research actually proves that **alcohol and tobacco are the true gateway drugs.**

How Drugs Are Taken (Route of Administration)

- *Oral ingestion (by mouth)*: The slowest way of getting drug effects; the drug has to pass through the digestive system and the liver before going to the brain.

- *Smoking*: The fastest way of getting drug effects; the drug enters capillaries in the lungs and goes directly to the brain.

- *Intravenous (IV) injection*: The second-fastest way to get drug effects (1 or 2 minutes). All injections depend on good hygiene to avoid serious infections and disease transmission.

- *Subcutaneous injection (skin-popping)*: An alternative to IV. There is a greater risk of infection and abscess this way. However, because it is a slower route to the brain and some of the drug is lost in tissue, there is a lower risk of overdose.

- *Intramuscular (IM) injection*: A common way of using some drugs—what most of us think of when we think "injection" (flu shots, for example).

- *Mucous membranes* in the nose, mouth, vagina, or rectum.

- *Topical or transdermal,* such as patches that are applied to the skin and then absorbed by capillaries close to the surface.

The Action of a Substance in the Brain

Of course the action of drugs in the brain is extremely complicated, but most drugs either stimulate or suppress the activity of neurotransmitters, the brain's chemical information system. They mimic, expand, lessen, bind to, or block these neurotransmitters.

Some of the Neurotransmitters Affected by Drugs

Dopamine: Responsible for fine-motor control and feelings of pleasure; influences the "addictive" potential of a drug because of the positive reinforcement of pleasurable feelings.

Norepinephrine (noradrenaline): The fight-or-flight chemical that arouses the brain/body when in danger; also facilitates alertness, learning, and memory processes.

GABA: The brain's sedative, it calms down brain activity much in the way the brakes work in a car. In other words, if norepinephrine is the gas pedal, GABA is the brakes.

Glutamate: A neurochemical that is widespread throughout the brain, glutamate is one of the primary neurotransmitters in the brain. It is excitatory, meaning that it stimulates nerves cells to fire, and is related to memory, learning, and attention. It regulates other neurotransmitters, serving as a stimulant to the actions of all neurotransmitters.

Serotonin: Regulates mood and aggression and is related to basic functions such as sex drive, appetite, and sleep. Serotonin influences some cognitive functions, including memory and learning.

Endorphins: The brain's endogenous (naturally occurring) opioids, they suppress pain (including emotional pain) and cause euphoria; opioid drugs mimic the action of endorphins by binding to the opioid receptors in the brain.

Anandamide and 2AG: Anandamide, whose name is derived from the Sanskrit word for "bliss," is one of the brain's endogenous cannabinoids. Anandamide is involved in regulating mood, memory, appetite, pain, cognition, and emotions. It also has effects in the peripheral nervous system involved in functions of the immune system. 2-Arachidonoylglycerol (2AG) was the second endogenous cannabinoid receptor identified. It is located in the central nervous system and regulates the effects of other cannabinoids. Cannabinoid receptors in the brain are located in the brain regions responsible for memory formation and coordination of movement. Cannabis and the cannabinoid system are extraordinarily complicated, and we are in the early days of understanding their complexity.

Acetylcholine: The main neurotransmitter in the body, it activates muscles and influences how the brain processes information, affecting arousal, attention, motivation, and mood. It regulates bodily functions such as heart rate, digestion, respiratory rate, pupil response, urination, sexual arousal, and reflexes such as coughing, sneezing, swallowing, and vomiting. The two major acetylcholine receptors are the nicotinic and muscarinic (think *Amanita muscaria,* a hallucinogenic mushroom).

Half-Life

Half-life is the time it takes for half of a substance to be eliminated from the body. In general, the shorter the half-life (short-acting as opposed to long-acting), the greater the misuse potential of the drug. This is because the "high" is lost very quickly, which leads to craving for more. Cocaine is a good example of this phenomenon; it is very short-acting, leading to a compulsion to use more and more of the drug.

BAC

The acronym *BAC* refers to blood alcohol concentration, also called blood alcohol level, measured in grams of alcohol per milliliter of blood: 0.08(%) is the legal limit for driving in the United States; 0.50(%) is enough to kill some people.

The Schedule of Drugs

In 1970, Congress enacted the Comprehensive Drug Abuse Prevention and Control Act, which established the Drug Enforcement Agency (DEA). This agency is a branch of the Department of Justice. This legislation, also called the Controlled Substances Act (CSA), requires that all persons who are involved in the manufacture and distribution of medicines/drugs register with the DEA. It also set up five "schedules," or categories, of drugs, supposedly based on a drug's potential for abuse and dependence and whether or not it was deemed to have any medical uses. Since then, every time a new recreational drug hits the streets, it is temporarily legal until the DEA finds out about it. Whether or not there are any studies proving that the drug has medical benefits or if it is addictive, it is usually "scheduled," always as a Schedule I drug. **The "schedule" that a drug is allocated to has nothing to do with its actual or potential medical benefits. It is a function of politics.**

- *Schedule I*: High abuse potential, no acceptable medical uses (for example, heroin, LSD, ecstasy, marijuana).
- *Schedule II*: High abuse potential; severe dependence but also accepted medical uses (opioids, barbiturates, amphetamines).

- *Schedule III*: Less abuse potential and only moderate dependence (primarily nonbarbiturate sedatives and nonamphetamine stimulants, and certain small amounts of narcotics).

- *Schedule IV*: Less abuse potential and limited dependence (antianxiety drugs, nonnarcotic pain relievers, some sedatives).

- *Schedule V*: Limited abuse potential (small amounts of codeine for use in cough syrups and antidiarrhea medicines).

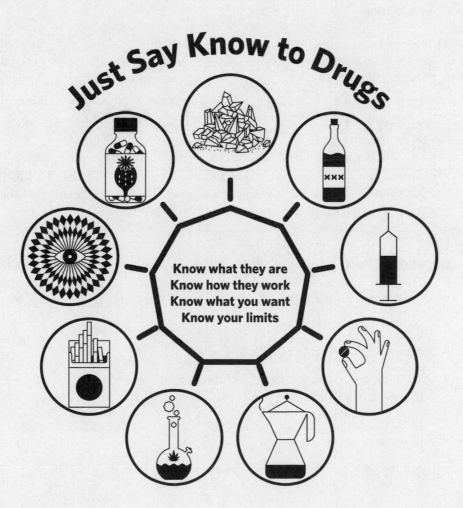

Just Say Know to Drugs

Know what they are
Know how they work
Know what you want
Know your limits

Alcohol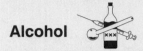

Ethanol is the only form of alcohol that can be consumed safely. *Methanol,* the product of home distilleries, is dangerous and can cause blindness. Alcohol might be the first intoxicant ever used. Early beer was more similar to a food than a beverage, and it is possible that early agriculture was intended to sustain sources of alcohol as well as other food. The use of wine as medicine has been recorded since the Sumerians wrote recipes for wine-based medicines in 2200 B.C. The Greek physician Hippocrates, who wrote "Do no harm," recommended wine as a disinfectant, a medicine, and an important part of a healthy diet. And the Jewish Talmud describes wine as "the foremost of all medicines."

How It Works

Alcohol affects more organ systems than any other drug: the liver, the heart, the stomach and digestive tract, the pancreas, and the brain. Alcohol passes through the digestive tract and is absorbed into the bloodstream through the intestines. It then passes through the liver prior to reaching the brain. Food and mixers dilute its effects and slow absorption. The first drink, however, passes straight from the stomach to the bloodstream without going through the intestine. This means a much more rapid effect for that first drink, especially if you drink on an empty stomach. In the brain, alcohol releases dopamine in moderate amounts. It increases the supply of GABA (the brain's natural sedative) and depresses the supply of glutamate (the brain's natural stimulant).

Beneficial Effects

- Social ritual and social "lubricant"

- Pleasure, euphoria

- Sedation, relaxation, anxiety reduction

- Disinhibition (loosens you up), which can either make you more at ease and friendlier or more aggressive, depending on what qualities have been suppressed by shyness or self-control.

- Pain relief

- Possible cardiovascular benefits (in moderate doses) due to lowering of LDL ("bad") cholesterol

Risks and Harmful Effects

Dependence, Tolerance, and Withdrawal

People develop tolerance to alcohol's psychoactive effects but very little to its psychomotor or physical effects. In other words, if you are a regular drinker, you may have to drink more to *feel* the intoxicating effects, but the more you drink, the more you will experience psychomotor impairment. This is why you may *think* you are able to drive if you have an increased tolerance to alcohol, but it is your BAC that determines your *actual* ability to drive.

Long-term, high-dose alcohol use causes physiological dependence. The withdrawal syndrome includes anxiety, depression or irritability, sweating, tremulousness, insomnia, seizure, and delirium tremens. Once alcohol's sedating effect has been removed, blood pressure, pulse, and heart rate rise, which can be dangerous. Delirium tremens (DTs) is an extreme version of withdrawal and constitutes a real medical emergency. If you experience severe shaking and sweating (how about seeing things?), you need medical attention—now!

Medical Risks

- Slowed heart rate and reflexes; loss of coordination.
- With long-term heavy use, cell loss in the hippocampus, where new memories are formed, causing problems with short-term memory, abstract thinking, problem solving, attention, and concentration.
- Alcohol crosses the blood–placenta barrier, putting fetuses at risk of birth defects.
- Nutritional deficiencies (B complex vitamins).
- Damage to blood vessels, nerve tissues, and brain (Wernicke-Korsakoff syndrome—permanent or acute cognitive impairment).
- Hypertension.
- Stomach distress and inflamed pancreas.
- Increased risk of certain cancers (head and neck, esophageal, liver, colorectal, breast).
- Lowered resistance to infection.
- Liver disease (fatty liver) that can progress to chronic alcoholic hepatitis or lethal cirrhosis.
- Alcohol poisoning due to respiratory depression, cardiac irregularities, coma, alcohol poisoning, overdose, or choking on vomit.

- Some East Asians produce an enzyme (ALD2★2) that is inefficient at breaking down acetaldehyde, a poisonous byproduct of alcohol, making them susceptible to flushing, headaches, nausea, vomiting, and heart palpitations.

Behavioral, Cognitive, and Psychological Risks

- Sedation, impaired concentration and memory.
- Depression or fluctuating moods.
- Blackouts or loss of memory while appearing to function "normally," with behaviors and interactions that are socially inappropriate ("drunk dialing," for example).
- Accidents and violence.
- Insomnia.

Drug Interactions

In combination with other drugs, the following effects can occur:

- Sedatives, anxiolytics (antianxiety meds like Valium), and narcotics (opioid pain medications): Increased sedation and risk of overdose.
- Antibiotics: Decreased effectiveness for some of these medicines.
- Antidepressants: Increase in sedative effects of tricyclics. No evidence of problems with SSRIs.
- Antipsychotics: Increased sedating effects.
- Antihistamines: Increased sedating effects.
- Acetaminophen: Should not be used by heavy drinkers because it taxes the liver.

Practicing Harm Reduction

"Less is more" (the same principle applies with a lot of drugs). You'll get more enjoyment and suffer fewer harms if you moderate your drinking. This means, first and foremost, not bingeing. When you drink a lot of alcohol at once, even if only once a week, it can cause more problems than regular moderate drinking.

- Drink lots of water and eat food before and while you're drinking. Drink a glass of water after each alcoholic drink—you will feel *much* better and you can still get tipsy.

- Limit your use of other drugs at the same time, especially sedatives or opioids, to reduce the risk of oversedation and overdose.

- Drink beer and wine rather than hard liquor.

- Count your drinks and pace yourself.

- Before drinking, make arrangements for transportation home.

- If a friend has had way too much to drink, don't just let him "sleep it off." He may just sleep himself to death, either by alcohol poisoning or choking on vomit. Stay with your friends until they sober up or at least until they throw up.

- When in doubt, call 911.

- *Times to avoid drinking or getting drunk*: when you're in a bad mood; if you have hepatitis or an otherwise compromised liver; on a date or at a party where you might end up in a sexually vulnerable situation; when driving; before having sex; when taking other sedating drugs.

Medication-Assisted Treatment

There are several medications that are used to help with alcohol problems.

- *Prevention*: Antabuse is prescribed to prevent people from drinking. It acts on liver enzymes so that even a small amount of alcohol causes intense discomfort (headache, vomiting). Larger amounts can lead to death. Other

What Is Moderate or Low-Risk Drinking?

For men: no more than 3–4 drinks a day, no more than 14 total per week.

For women: no more than 3 drinks a day, no more than 7–8 total per week.

For older adults: less than the above. As people age, our levels of ALD2, which metabolizes alcohol, diminishes.

If you stay within these guidelines, you have only a 2% chance of developing an alcohol problem in the future.

If you exceed these guidelines two or more times a week, you have a 50% chance!

Sources: www.rethinkingdrinking.niaaa.nih.gov, www.moderation.org, *and* www.moderatedrinking.com.

medications are meant to either decrease cravings or block the pleasurable effects of alcohol.

- *Reduction*: Naltrexone (which comes in a long-acting injectable called Vivitrol) is the most commonly used medication and is effective for some people, but it is not, by any means, a stand-alone treatment. There is increasing evidence that the way we typically prescribe naltrexone in the United States every day is not as effective as the Sinclair Method used in some European countries. In this variation, you take the medicine only when you plan to drink. The pleasure of alcohol and the desire to drink are reduced at the time that you are drinking, and people typically drink less. This immediate feedback is thought to have a more potent effect on your wish to drink on future days.

- *Detoxification*: Benzodiazepines such as Valium or Librium are used for a few days, prescribed either on an outpatient basis or in an inpatient detox program. If you don't have access to medications or a detox program, and you become too tremulous or have a seizure history, a little alcohol will stop the withdrawal process. In fact, you can detox yourself by drinking ever-decreasing amounts of alcohol. Heavy drinkers might find this discipline challenging, but a little less alcohol is better than dangerous withdrawal, at least in the short term, until you can get medical help.

Cannabis

Marijuana, hashish, wax, oil: *Cannabis* is the general botanical name of the plant that produces marijuana. Cannabis falls into no drug category; it has many different properties and effects—*industrial, medicinal, social,* and *perception-altering.* There are three main types of cannabis—sativa, indica, and hemp (a variety of sativa that has little psychoactive effect). Hemp has been used for thousands of years. It can be refined into paper, textiles, biodegradable plastics, paint, insulation, biofuel, food, and animal feed. Psychoactive cannabis has been used medicinally for thousands of years. Cannabis is smoked, vaporized, eaten (in cookies, brownies, candy, butter, even gummy bears!), and made into salves and lotions.

Typically these days, marijuana has a THC concentration of 16–40%, compared to the 1–8% concentration in the marijuana imported from Mexico in the 1960s and '70s. The concentration of THC can go up to 85% for "wax."

Generally, by those not directly involved in carrying out the War on Drugs, marijuana is considered the safest of all recreational drugs, and its medical uses far outweigh its problems as an intoxicant. At the time of publication, medical use and/

or possession of small amounts for personal consumption has been legalized in more than half of U.S. states.

How It Works

There are 400 active ingredients in the cannabis plant, with THC (tetrahydrocannabinol) being the most potent. CBD (cannabidiol) is another important ingredient. It is not psychoactive; instead, it has anti-inflammatory properties and is used for pain and muscle spasms.

The receptors in the brain that respond to marijuana were only discovered in 1990. THC receptors are found mostly in the hippocampus, which controls new memory formation (learning); in the cerebellum and basal ganglia, which coordinate fine-motor movements; and in the nucleus acumbens, which contains dopamine. There are few cannabis receptors in the brainstem, which controls vital functions such as respiration, so there is no risk of overdose or death. For occasional users, THC can be detected in the urine up to 20 hours after use and up to several weeks in regular users. It accumulates in the tissues of the liver, kidneys, spleen, and testes and is stored in fatty tissue and released slowly. THC crosses the blood–placenta barrier.

THC's psychoactive effects last a few hours. If smoked, it goes from lungs to heart to brain in a few seconds, peaks in 10–20 minutes, and lasts up to a couple of hours. When eaten, it goes through the liver first. Its effects may not be felt for an hour, but the high lasts longer because of the slower route, and eating it is more likely to induce a hallucinatory experience than smoking.

Cannabis is very sensitive to set and setting, more so than most other drugs. Some people experience relaxation and sedation, others stimulation, still others anxiety and paranoia. It depends on one's preexisting mood, mental health, and expectations as well as on where and with whom one uses.

Beneficial Effects

Cannabis has many, many medical and social uses. Here are just a few.

Psychological/Cognitive

- Sensation of brilliance and creativity; ability to freely explore interesting and new trains of thought
- Feelings of openness, relaxation, lightness, and hilarity
- Greater connection between mind and body, and with other people

- Reduced anxiety, stress, and aggression
- Reduced feelings of depression
- Altered perception of time

Medical

Various medical benefits can be gained from smoking/vaporizing, oral ingestion, or use of salves and creams:

- Increases appetite and decreases nausea (useful for people with AIDS and chemotherapy patients).
- Reduces eye pressure from glaucoma.
- Relaxes muscles; useful for multiple sclerosis and other disorders that cause muscle spasticity.

Cannabis can also be used to treat the following conditions:

- Seizures
- Migraines
- Chronic pain
- Asthma (when vaporized or taken orally)

Risks and Harmful Effects

Cannabis is the least harmful of all recreational drugs. The current consensus among scientists is that marijuana does not cause serious psychiatric or medical problems in the vast majority of people who use it. Nor is there risk of overdose, as it does not affect the brainstem, where vital functions are regulated.

Dependence, Tolerance, and Withdrawal

Tolerance develops to cannabis (and some control can be gained over effects on coordination and concentration—but not enough to operate a car!); it develops more rapidly in heavy users. Withdrawal is generally mild, with irritability, restlessness, insomnia, bad dreams, sweating, headaches, and mild nausea possible for a short time.

Research indicates that the rate of developing a substance use disorder with regular use does not increase over time. This means that about 9% of regular users will develop problems, but the rate doesn't rise if you've been using for 3 years or 30! Marijuana is thought to have low misuse potential, due to its relatively mild activation of dopamine. Psychological dependence can develop in regular users, and many people struggle to control or stop their marijuana use.

Physiological

- Impairs attention, concentration, and reaction time (to some extent, these can be relearned while under the influence).

- Drowsiness, dry mouth, dizziness (these are generally uncomfortable but not necessarily harmful).

- Blocks airflow in heavy smokers, contains some of the same carcinogens as tobacco, and can cause coughing and upper respiratory problems.

- Researchers disagree about whether cannabis lowers testosterone levels and sperm count, or suppresses the hormone necessary for the implanting of fertilized eggs. But long-term use does seem to have the effect of suppressing the production of hormones that regulate the reproductive systems of men and women.

- Increased heart rate for up to 3 hours and lowered blood pressure may increase the chance of heart attack. Older people and those with heart problems may be at higher risk.

- The evidence of any impact on infants (lower birth weight) is confounded by the often accompanying use of alcohol and tobacco.

Psychological/Cognitive

- Anxiety, confusion, paranoia, and panic.

- Difficulty with short-term memory is common while high (see the next page for a longer discussion of memory).

- Disrupts linear thinking, which is usually experienced as pleasant.

- The so-called "amotivational syndrome," referring to the loss of motivation to set goals or accomplish tasks, has been pretty well disproven by research, but we observe a lack of motivation in a subset of people who are heavy users. They think their pot smoking has contributed to disorganization, low self-esteem, and a lack of motivation and impaired their intimate relationships. They feel these problems "snuck up" on them over time.

- Feelings of being detached from oneself can be disturbing to some (and pleasurable to others).

Behavioral

- Accidents while driving, and psychomotor retardation that can last for at least 24 hours after using. The idea that one can drive better when stoned is being disproved over and over again as more states move to legalize cannabis.

Memory

One way of approaching the research on cannabis and memory is to distinguish between acute, residual, and chronic effects.

- *Acute intoxication*: New memory formation (learning) is impaired. Mental flexibility and problem-solving ability may be impaired in heavy users.

- *Residual effects*: These effects are generally caused by the long-acting nature of marijuana. Once the intoxicating effects have worn off (4–6 hours), THC remains in the brain and in body tissues for 48 hours or longer. Thus the ability to form new memories may be impaired for 2 days after using. This also means that even if one uses only every couple of days, the brain is never clear of some THC and its effects on memory formation and problem solving.

- *Chronic effects*: There are several studies suggesting that long-term use results in decreases in abstract thinking, problem solving (less mental flexibility—people made the same mistakes over and over in trying to solve problems), the ability to process information quickly, and short-term memory. Much more research is needed, as the sample size of the studies is probably not large enough to give us a full picture of how many chronic users will suffer these memory deficits.

Use by Adolescents: Age as a Mediating Factor

This is where the research, the beliefs, and the debate become more complicated, but also more important. Teenagers' estimate of the risks of using marijuana are very low, their parents are worried that any use will stunt their growth, and the research can offer some solace or support to both groups. Studies need to be conducted using much larger numbers of subjects, but there is a body of literature suggesting that early onset and then regular use of cannabis can cause significant problems with learning and some other cognitive functions. Use before the age of 15 seems to interfere with the development of visual scanning, and regular use before the age of 18 is related to a decrease in problem-solving ability, memory formation, and mental flexibility. When comparing heavy users who have been using for over 8 years, the only predictor of cognitive problems was age of first use.

In contrast, a recent long-range study showed *no difference* between heavy users and nonusers in physical or mental health effects.

The key seems to be the role of cannabis on the developing hippocampus. Teenagers who use show an increase in acute memory problems but a *decrease* in anxiety reactions. So while they are not performing as well as they might, they are not receiving internal negative feedback about their cognitive deficits.

In our opinion, there is some reason to be concerned about using cannabis with any regularity before the age of 18. Here's the bottom line:

- Cannabinoids sometimes remain in the brain and body long after the intoxication wears off.

- The brain develops rapidly between the ages of 13 and 19.

- Continued use into adulthood may prevent social, psychological, or cognitive problems from being overcome.

Practicing Harm Reduction

According to the most recent studies, the major risks for adults can be avoided by limiting the quantity and frequency of use and by limiting the amount of smoke inhaled. The recent use of vaporizers counteracts the dangers of smoke inhalation, as does the choice of "edibles." Using lower-potency products is a good idea if you are going to be using multiple times a week (or daily). In terms of medical use, there is some reason to believe that finding the correct dose and the optimum schedule of use increases the benefits, while overusing can actually negate some of the medical benefits. For teenagers, once-a-week, low-potency, vaporized marijuana is probably safe, but we can't prove it. For people who are expecting regular-grade cannabis but use much more potent products and find that they are higher than expected, this can lead to panic and unnecessary hospital visits.

Finally, cannabis is often a harm reduction remedy for people who are trying to reduce or stop the use of other drugs. Cannabis has helped many of our clients reduce or quit alcohol and opioids.

Sedatives/Hypnotics and Anxiolytics

Chloral hydrate; barbiturates (Nembutal, Seconal, Amytal); **benzodiazepines**: Valium, Librium, Rohypnol (roofies), Ativan, Dalmane, Ambien, Klonopin,

Restoril, Versed, Xanax; **GHB:** gamma-hydroxybutyrate (Liquid X, Easy Lay, Grievous Bodily Harm); **GBL** (gamma-butyrolactone), which converts to GHB when ingested.

The term *sedative/hypnotic* refers to the combined sedating and sleep-inducing effects of these drugs (*hypnosis* comes from the name of the Greek god of sleep). *Anxiolytic* refers to the antianxiety effects of these drugs, the reason many were developed. Chloral hydrate was the first of these drugs, developed in the mid-1800s for use in treating insomnia. A few drops in whiskey was called a Mickey Finn. Unfortunately, effective as it was, it irritated the stomach. Barbiturates, developed in 1903, were so effective for sedation, anesthesia, and seizures (they depress electrical activity in the brain) that 2,500 types were synthesized. All barbiturates depress vital functions, especially respiration, so overdosing is easy, and they became the most common method of suicide in the United States. Benzodiazepines, first developed in 1957, became a safer substitute. They too cause sedation but without effects on vital functions such as breathing and heart rate, making them the safest of the anxiolytic medications. Methaqualone was developed in the 1970s as another alternative but became a recreational drug of abuse (Quaaludes). When reports of overdoses started appearing, it was made a Schedule I drug in 1984 and is no longer manufactured in the United States. Rohypnol (roofies) is most often associated with date rape, and it also creates amnesia surrounding whatever is experienced while intoxicated. GHB is a naturally occurring substance that is similar to GABA. It is used in clubs and raves as a party drug and is sometimes associated with date rape, because it creates sedation and amnesia for the experience.

How They Work

Sedatives/hypnotics/anxiolytics are central nervous system depressants. Barbiturates act on the reticular activating system, which induces sleep, slows respiration as well as heart rate, and lowers blood pressure. They also increase the activity of GABA, which slows down brain activity by reducing electrical activity). Benzodiazepines, the most commonly used antianxiety drugs nowadays, increase the function of GABA only indirectly. They induce sedation and relaxation without inhibiting respiration or significantly slowing heartbeat. Different kinds of benzodiazepines have different half-lives (length of action), so some are more useful for sleep (Klonopin, for example), whereas others are useful for panic attacks or short-lived anxiety-producing situations such as flying (Xanax, for example). Still others are so sedating as well as short-acting (Versed) that they are used only during surgery.

Beneficial Effects

Medical

- Sedation, sleep, anesthetic antiseizure, alcohol detox.

Psychological

- Reduce anxiety, panic.

- Relaxation, some mild euphoria.

- Feeling of being at ease, including in social interactions.

- Sometimes used in combination with stimulants to decrease some of the negative effects stimulants produce, such as muscle tension.

Risks and Harmful Effects

Risks range from serious dangers to harms that are mostly just uncomfortable.

Dependence, Tolerance, and Withdrawal

Tolerance and physical dependence develop rapidly with barbiturates and can lead to fatal overdose, preceded by drowsiness, nausea, headache, loss of reflexes, loss of consciousness, and suppression of breathing. They are especially dangerous when mixed with alcohol or other sedative drugs. Benzodiazepines do not, by themselves, result in fatal overdoses; the deaths that have been studied were related to use in combination with alcohol and other central nervous system depressant drugs such as opioids. For example, 80% of GHB deaths have involved alcohol.

These drugs have potentially dangerous withdrawal symptoms similar to alcohol. Benzodiazepines tend to produce significant tolerance and dependence only with high-dose, long-term use. They should be discontinued under medical supervision to prevent serious withdrawal symptoms, which can lead to death. GHB also has potentially dangerous withdrawal symptoms, though many people do not use it regularly enough to develop tolerance and dependence.

Medical Risks

- Lightheadedness, vertigo, drowsiness, slurred speech, and muscle incoordination.

- Accidents and falls.

- Long-term use of benzodiazepines can inhibit short-term memory and new learning and may also cause amnesia (especially Rohypnol and GHB). Recent research points to an increased risk of developing Alzheimer's disease with regular use, even at therapeutic doses.

Psychological/Behavioral

- "Disinhibition" (much like alcohol): risk of errors in judgment, emotional swings, putting yourself in dangerous sexual situations.
- Some people have what is called a "paradoxical reaction" and become agitated instead of calm (especially older adults).

Drug Interactions

The major danger with these is mixing them with other central nervous system depressants (alcohol, opioids, ketamine, and other sedatives). Such mixing dramatically increases the risk of overdose.

Practicing Harm Reduction

Again, the motto is "Less is more." It is really tempting to overuse these drugs, especially benzodiazepines, because they make you feel good and rarely have unpleasant side effects. Doing them only occasionally is the best way to enjoy them and avoid problems. Always start with a small dose and wait 30 to 60 minutes before taking more. Remember, the dose can last up to 4 hours.

Mixing these various drugs, because they belong to the same class, is not a good idea, for all of the reasons above. If you do take these drugs to counteract stimulants that you are using, be aware that you will not be able to feel the full effect of the cocaine or speed so easily, and you might be tempted to use more than your body can handle. It's best to wait until the end of your speed or cocaine use to take these drugs. That way, you're not adding a drug that will confuse the picture.

As with alcohol, don't drive or operate machinery when using any of these drugs, unless you're using regular, appropriate amounts prescribed for anxiety or for a seizure disorder.

Opioids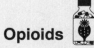

Opium is derived from the sticky resin in the seed pod of the opium poppy. It contains two active ingredients, **morphine** and **codeine**. **Laudanum** is opium mixed with alcohol. **Hydromorphone** (Dilaudid), **oxymorphone** (Opana), **oxycodone** (Percodan), and **hydrocodone** (Vicodin) are chemically modified substances derived from morphine or codeine. **Oxycodone hydrochloride controlled release** (Oxycontin) is a time-release chemical modification of codeine. **Heroin** is a chemical modification of morphine to speed absorption in the brain.

Meperidine (Demerol), **methadone, buprenorphine,** and **fentanyl** are synthetic opioids that are not derived from the opium poppy. Opioids vary greatly in potency, including, from most to least potent: fentanyl, Dilaudid, heroin, morphine, Demerol, and codeine.

The earliest references to opium come from Babylonia/Assyria 4,000 years ago. Morpheus, the Greek god of dreams, is often depicted with poppies in his hands. Opium has been a major ingredient of many tonics and medicines, including "Mrs. Winslow's Soothing Syrup," a teething formula for babies, and paregoric, also used for teething babies and for diarrhea. Chinese immigrants introduced the smoking of opium to the United States, where it became popular and then became the first banned drug in this country in 1906. Opioids have been controlled substances since 1914. Today only heroin is a Schedule I drug (unavailable for any medical use)—even though it was developed and marketed as a medicine by the Bayer company in 1898, 2 years before they marketed aspirin.

Opioid overdose increased 200% between 2000 and 2014. There were 47,000 drug overdose deaths in the United States in 2014, 61% of them attributable to opioid drugs. The increase between 2013 and 2014 is partly attributable to increased availability of fentanyl, including illegally manufactured fentanyl. Various measures have been taken to reduce the misuse of prescription medications. Oxycontin has been reformulated to prevent injection. Unfortunately, the reformulation of Opana (oxymorphone) to prevent snorting that drug led many to inject it in Scott County, Indiana, causing an infectious disease outbreak in 2015, as distribution of clean syringes was illegal until after the outbreak, which led to hundreds of new cases of HIV and hepatitis C infection. *Many drug deaths would be avoided if there were no stigma and secrecy surrounding drug use and naloxone was freely available to everyone in the event of an overdose.*

How They Work

In the brain, opioids initially release dopamine, especially if injected, then bind to endorphin and enkephalin receptor sites. Endorphins regulate mood, digestion, body temperature, and breathing, and create calm when the organism is under stress. Enkephalins communicate messages in parts of the brain that process pain sensation and regulate breathing, and in parts where the reward system (dopamine) operates. The main opioid receptor (called the mu receptor) provides analgesia, euphoria, and respiratory depression. Opioids also constrict pupils, called "pinprick pupils," which is not actually harmful.

Regular opioid use shuts down production of the brain's endogenous opioid system. Research suggests that the longer one uses opioids, the less likely it is that these internal opioids will regenerate, but this long-term effect remains unclear. Another possible explanation for dependence on opioids is that many people who become dependent on opioids do so because they never had good enough endorphin systems—perhaps due to early-life trauma—and therefore opioid drugs become a very effective way of self-medicating.

Opioids are easily absorbed by many routes of administration: heroin can be used in any way; pills can be swallowed or crushed and snorted or injected. This varies for each type of opioid because of the chemical composition of the pill. How fast they get to the brain depends on the particular drug and the route of administration—for example, fentanyl is most impactful because of its potency. The user generally doesn't experience a rush if the opioid is taken orally. Shooting opioids results in a "rush" of euphoria from dopamine, and many people use this method just because of that rush. Effects after the initial euphoria last 4–6 hours, except for methadone (12–24 hours) and fentanyl (1 hour).

Beneficial Effects

Opioids are unparalleled in their medical applications for analgesia (decreased pain sensation), cough suppression, antidiarrheal use, and sedation. Their psychological effects include:

- Euphoria, pleasant floating sensation, dreamlike state.
- Soothing sense of warmth, safety, and well-being.
- Blunting of emotional pain and worry; feeling of separation from worries and pain.
- Softening feelings of depression.
- Relaxation; can enhance enjoyable feelings with friends (at lower doses; at higher doses, one tends to drift off).

Risks and Harmful Effects

Opioids are generally benign substances and cause no direct damage to the body. They have given humans great benefits and have also caused an enormous amount of suffering. Some of this suffering has occurred from overuse of the drug, polluted supplies, and poor hygiene. Much of the suffering, though, has been due to the erratic legal and social sanctions regarding these drugs as well as the changing attitudes of physicians.

Dependence, Tolerance, and Withdrawal

Tolerance develops to the euphoric and analgesic effects, which means higher doses can be tolerated the longer one uses. However, tolerance does *not* develop to respiratory depression, constipation, or pinpoint pupils. Tolerance is partly setting dependent, meaning that one's tolerance can be different (higher or lower) depending on where and with whom one is using. This variability is possibly due to the body's response of "readying" itself to counter the effects of a drug, a process that is initiated by the cues in one's familiar using environment. It is possible that people who use opioids for intense or chronic pain, not for recreation, do not develop tolerance to the analgesic effects as quickly as those who use recreationally. Cross-tolerance develops with all opioid drugs.

Physiological dependence due to tolerance causes a withdrawal syndrome of flu-like symptoms: cramps, chills, sweating, nausea, increased pain sensation, insomnia, increased heart rate, restlessness, diarrhea, and dysphoria (depression). The worst effects occur from 24 to 72 hours after last use and can last up to a week. For several weeks or months after stopping, people are more sensitive to pain and depressed feelings.

Medical Risks

- Overdose: **Opioids in combination with other drugs that depress respiration, such as alcohol, benzodiazepines, GHB, or barbiturates, can be deadly.** Overdose is due primarily to respiratory depression or oversedation, which can lead to coma. Warning signs are (1) respiration lower than 12 breaths per minute, (2) unconsciousness or extreme drowsiness, (3) unresponsiveness to pain, (4) turning blue in the face. Overdoses can happen to naïve users who take a dose larger than their tolerance can handle; to regular users when a stronger batch of heroin hits the streets or it has been "cut" with fentanyl; to regular users who use in a different location; or to former users who have quit (perhaps in jail or rehab), then return to using their usual dose.

- Nausea and vomiting. If you are high, vomiting could put you in danger of choking.

- Constipation.

Risks Due to Use Practices Largely Driven by the War on Drugs

- HIV, hepatitis, other blood–borne diseases.

- Vein damage due to injecting particles or using large/damaged needles.

- Abscesses and other bacterial infections including endocarditis, inflammation of the lining of the heart, caused by contaminants.

- Poor nutrition.

Drug Interactions

- Mixing opioids and opioid drugs with other central nervous system depressants (alcohol, benzodiazepines, barbiturates, GHB, and ketamine) increases the risk of overdose.

- Mixing with stimulants masks the effects of opioids, so you might take more than you intend of either. Stimulants, especially cocaine, greatly increase overdose risk.

Practicing Harm Reduction

Much of the harm caused by opioid use could be prevented by public health interventions:

- Making clean syringes available (so people wouldn't have to share their "works," thus spreading HIV and other infections).

- Teaching people safer injection techniques (including how to test their dose for potency).

- Teaching people how to perform rescue breathing.

- Making Narcan available more readily.

- Offering a wider range of treatment options for those who want to quit or cut back, like methadone and buprenorphine replacement.

- Opening safe injection facilities like InSite in Vancouver or drug consumption rooms (where any drug can be used) to guarantee safe use in a medically supervised environment.

In the absence of these needed services, here are some tips:

- If new, clean syringes aren't available, follow the bleach guidelines (clean syringe and *all* works with bleach, then water, three times, then a final rinse with water).

- Test your dose of heroin—try a small amount to test for potency, then shoot the rest. Remember that different batches of heroin have different potencies and are different in different parts of the country.

- It is not wise to crush up pills and shoot them—yeah, we know, sometimes that's all that's available—but pills contain a lot of fillers that are OK in your stomach but can cause damage to veins and serious damage to the smaller blood vessels in your lungs. Even the best "cottons" might not filter out all the gunk. Filter more than once.

- Consider not shooting. Snorting may not get you off as quickly and you may waste a little, but it might work better for you in terms of your overall health. Smoking is a rapid way to use many opioids and carries little of the risks of shooting. Or consider pills. You generally don't feel a rush this way, but it's safer.

- Beware of pills that have acetaminophen (Tylenol) in them. This drug is hard on your liver, so taking large quantities can be dangerous, especially if you drink a lot or have hepatitis C.

Medication-Assisted Treatment

- *Overdose—naloxone* (Narcan) blocks opioid receptors and reverses drug effects. It acts quickly and can be administered by injection, nasal spray, or an auto-injector (like an EpiPen for allergic reactions). Naloxone is now legal to buy without a prescription in many states.

- *Deterrence—naltrexone* (ReVia) also blocks opioid receptors so you can't get high, but it is taken orally, so it acts more slowly and is not useful for emergency use to interrupt overdose. It is not effective for many people, and some report that it makes them feel more depressed.

- *Withdrawal—clonidine* (Catapres) lowers heart rate and eases restlessness.

- *Detoxification—methadone* or *buprenorphine* is used in outpatient settings for detox.

- *Substitution—methadone* and *buprenorphine* are also excellent medicines for long-term drug substitution. Unfortunately, methadone puts you into a "system" of care in federally controlled clinics rather than, as with buprenorphine, under the care of a private physician who can make decisions based on less restrictive federal guidelines.

Synthetic Opioids

Kratom, Krypton, Krokodil: Kratom and Krypton are both opioid analogues but from very different sources. Kratom is an herbal drug from a plant that has been used medicinally for thousands of years in Southeast Asia. Its main chemical is mitragynine, which acts on the mu opioid receptor. At low doses it provides stimulant effects, and at higher doses it causes typical opioid reactions: euphoria and relaxation.

Krypton is a combination of herbal kratom with the active metabolite of tramadol, a potent opioid agonist. This combination results in a substance that is twice as potent as tramadol itself and has been known to cause a significant number of overdoses. Then there is Krypton Kratom, a mix of caffeine and the active metabolite of tramadol that people can mistake for Kratom.

Krokodil (desomorphone) is an opioid made from codeine pills. It was developed primarily in Russia as a substitute for heroin, which had become very hard to find and very expensive due to the government's crackdown on heroin imports and use. But codeine pills were still readily available over the counter, so people used solvents and the phosphorus from matches to synthesize the drug desomorphone. Because it is both caustic and often highly contaminated from being made in unsanitary conditions, this drug causes severe tissue inflammation that often leads to the skin and muscle sloughing off from injection sites and the limbs developing gangrene. This drug is not known to be used in the United States despite some recent media hysteria.

Major Stimulants

Cocaine—*leaf* is chewed in the Andes; *powder*: cocaine hydrochloride, a crystalline distillate of coca leaves, snorted or dissolved for injection; *crack*: cocaine boiled with bicarbonate of soda to precipitate the cocaine base and smoked; **ephedrine**—active ingredient of the Chinese herb ma huang; **amphetamines**—a family of ephedrine-based stimulants (brand name Benzedrine) and **dextroamphetamine** (Dexedrine, Adderall); **methamphetamine**—a chemical derivative of amphetamine (speed, ice, or crystal), brand names Desoxyn, Methedrine; **nonamphetamine stimulants**—methylphenidate (Ritalin), prescribed for attention deficit disorder, and modafinil (Provigil), which promotes wakefulness without the central nervous system effects of other stimulants; **khat**—mild stimulant from a leafy plant in East Africa and southern Saudi Arabia; cathinone is the active ingredient; methcathinone is a synthetic form of khat.

There are many other plants and seeds that have stimulant properties and are widely used in local areas around the world. Betel seeds (India) can be chewed, and yohimbine, from the bark of an African tree, has been used as an intoxicant, an aphrodisiac, and a medicine. A lot of the so-called designer drugs are stimulants. More about that later.

Cocaine is a central nervous system stimulant, a vasoconstrictor, and a local anesthetic, and was an ingredient in the original Coca-Cola. It is the active ingredient derived from the coca leaf found in the rainforests and fields of the upper slopes of the Andes and used there for at least 5,000 years. The coca leaf contains no more than 2% cocaine, whereas refined cocaine is almost 100% pure and crack cocaine, when not purposely cut, is about 75% pure cocaine. It takes about 250 pounds of coca leaves to produce 1 pound of cocaine.

Ephedras are plants that grow mostly in desert areas. Ephedrine, the active ingredient of the Chinese plant ma huang, has been used for 5,000 years to treat asthma, because it stimulates the nerves that dilate bronchioles. In the United States, the Mormons, who are not allowed to use caffeine or take other intoxicating drugs, discovered a bush containing ephedra and learned to make a stimulant tea from its leaves, commonly referred to as "Mormon tea."

Amphetamines and their derivatives are synthetic forms of ephedrine. However, ephedrine does not have the psychoactive properties of amphetamines. Methamphetamine, the most popular form for recreational use, is a chemical derivative that allows quicker passage across the blood–brain barrier. Amphetamine was developed and used for treatment of asthma and as a decongestant, for alertness and focus, weight loss, and ADHD.

There are many nonamphetamine stimulants, including herbal varieties and medicinal pharmaceutical drugs. Methcathinone is the synthetic form of khat, which has been chewed in Yemen and other Middle Eastern countries for centuries. Heavily used in the former Soviet Union in the 1970s and '80s, methcathinone once represented 20% of all illicit drug use in that country.

How They Work

Stimulants increase the amount of norepinephrine in the brain. Norepinephrine is the neurotransmitter that controls the fight-or-flight response and is a part of the emergency response system. It controls the sympathetic nervous system, increasing heart rate and respiration, constricting blood vessels, and increasing blood pressure—all necessary to the emergency response system, but creating the symptoms of chronic stress if activated on a regular basis.

Cocaine and amphetamine also dramatically increase levels of dopamine and serotonin, more than any other recreational drug, making them the most "reward-ing" of all drugs. They work in slightly different ways: amphetamine more closely resembles the norepinephrine and dopamine molecules. It actively releases the neu-rotransmitters into the synapse as well as blocking their reuptake, whereas cocaine only blocks reuptake, making more of our natural supplies of dopamine and nor-epinephrine available for use (the same effect that SSRI antidepressants have on serotonin).

The most dramatic difference is the duration of effect: cocaine's effects last from a few minutes to an hour, while amphetamine's effects can be felt for up to 12 hours.

Stimulants increase heart rate, blood pressure, body temperature, and respira-tion. Increased blood flow prolongs erection and delays ejaculation. Dilated bron-chioles allow for more oxygen to enter the lungs. Suppressed appetite makes stimu-lants useful as diet medicines.

Beneficial Effects

Medical

Stimulants are used in the treatment of

- ADHD, in both children and adults.
- Obesity.
- Narcolepsy.
- Nasal congestion.

Psychological/Cognitive

- Euphoria, energy, mood enhancement.
- Focus—sense of sharpness.
- Counteract the flattening effects of some antipsychotic medications for schizo-phrenia and mood-stabilizing medications for bipolar disorder (manic–depression).

Behavioral

- Partying.
- Sexual appetite and performance (unless overused, when erectile dysfunction sets in).

Risks and Harmful Effects

Dependence, Tolerance, and Withdrawal

Cocaine and methamphetamine are compelling due to a euphoric "rush" from the release of dopamine. This effect makes them intensely pleasurable and reinforces their continued use. There has always been debate about whether stimulants cause physiological dependence. Suffice it to say that they create enough changes in the functioning of the norepinephrine, serotonin, and dopamine systems that they produce powerful cravings and other reactions that make up what is basically a tolerance and withdrawal syndrome.

Tolerance develops to stimulant effects, making it more difficult to get high, but reverses with a few days of abstinence. Repetitive motor activity and paranoia get more exaggerated with long-term use. Withdrawal or crashing creates symptoms of depression and anhedonia (inability to feel pleasure), probably due to a deficiency of dopamine, which leads to craving, irritability, and possibly aggressiveness for up to several months. Exhaustion is also experienced, probably due to a depletion of norepinephrine and lack of sleep during a long cocaine or speed run.

Medical Risks

- Headaches, nausea, vomiting, chest pains, dizziness.

- Erectile dysfunction and delayed ejaculation (constricts blood vessels in penis).

- With heavy, prolonged use, repetitive movements that can be bizarre or self-destructive, such as skin picking.

- Because they release dopamine, stimulants also can cause psychotic symptoms in people who use a lot, or in vulnerable people (those with schizophrenia, for example). Paranoia, hallucinations, and delusions may sometimes lead to violence as the person tries to protect him- or herself from "attacks by enemies." These symptoms usually resolve with discontinued use.

- Mood swings from euphoric to depressed.

- Snorting can damage the interior of the nose, causing lesions.

- Regular use restricts blood flow to the capillaries, causing gum deterioration.

- Lack of moisture in the mouth results in dental cavities.

- Regular use often leads to poor nutrition (stimulants interrupt digestion as well as interfering with appetite).

- Chronic activation of the fight-or-flight response can impair immune function due to repeated release of stress hormones (cortisol, for example).

- Poor nutrition and fatigue from speed use can further compromise a weakened immune system.

- Overdose—increased heart rate can cause irregular heart rhythm and extremely elevated blood pressure, leading to stroke or heart attack. If stimulants are used at *closely spaced intervals,* the effects on the brain diminish long before the body eliminates the drugs, so one can accumulate toxic levels of drug. It is also possible to overdose with a single heavy dose. Speedballs (a combination of speed or cocaine and heroin) reduce sensation of both the opioids and the stimulant, thus increasing the chance of overdose.

- Long-term use can lead to atherosclerosis (fatty buildup in blood vessels) or damage to the heart due to lack of oxygen.

- Seizures can occur when blood levels of stimulant are high: emergency room admissions for seizures are checked for stimulant use when the patient has no seizure history.

- Ephedrine can be toxic to the cardiovascular system at two to three times the recommended dose (often recommended for recreational drug effect).

- There is some evidence that long-term methamphetamine use causes a complete breakdown in the serotonin system, which results not only in depressed mood, but dysregulation of all the other brain chemicals as well. This system is slow to recover and may be permanently damaged in some people. Methamphetamine causes actual damage to dopamine and norepinephrine neurons as well: nerve endings are cut back, causing deficits in the amount of these neurotransmitters that is available; longer-term connections to movement and mood disorders are unknown at this point.

Drug Interactions

The most serious interaction occurs between cocaine and alcohol. When they are used together, the liver enzymes that metabolize the two drugs combine to form an active metabolite (cocaethylene). This metabolite is stronger than cocaine and lasts much longer, thus contributing to more overdoses and a more serious withdrawal if a person is dependent on both drugs. Combining stimulants will enhance and exaggerate the toxic effects of each.

Practicing Harm Reduction

- Don't dose on the high—there is still stimulant left in your body. If you have to take more the same day, dose on the half-life (the time it takes for half the drug to leave your body): 2 to 4 hours for cocaine, 8 to 12 hours for speed.

- Dilute when possible: if you snort, snort with water—it's easier on the nose.

- Maintain regular sleep and eating habits.

- Try not to combine stimulants, either with other stimulants, which potentiate the effects, or with depressants, which mask what's happening to your body and mind.

- Try not to use to get through your usual activities of the day. In other words, use purposefully—know why you use and use for only that purpose.

- Use antipsychotic medications to treat stimulant psychosis; these should be withdrawn after symptoms disappear.

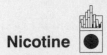

Nicotine

Cigarettes, cigars, pipes, hookah, chew, snuff: Nicotine belongs to its own drug class, although it has many stimulant properties. Most people, after an initial period of coughing from the smoke, enjoy the effects of nicotine. In high concentrations nicotine is a toxic substance. Sixty milligrams of nicotine would be enough to kill an adult. Cigarettes contain from half a milligrams to 2 milligrams, however, and only 20% of that amount is ingested while smoking. A little more is ingested by chewing or snuff.

How It Works

When smoked, nicotine goes immediately from lungs to blood to brain, where it stimulates acetylcholine neurotransmitters, otherwise known as *nicotinic receptors*. These release dopamine and increase activity in brain regions associated with memory and physical movement. The release of dopamine and the speed of action in the brain make nicotine very reinforcing. The effect peaks in 10 minutes or less, and nicotine has a half-life of 20 minutes. Nicotine elevates heart rate and blood pressure. It also suppresses appetite, for unclear reasons.

Beneficial Effects

Nicotine, in and of itself, is not a harmful drug at low (nontoxic) doses. It has several actual and potential benefits:

- Energy.
- Relaxation without dulling the senses.
- Nicotine has shown greater potential than amphetamines to enhance

memory, concentration, and focus. It is being researched for use to treat both ADHD and Alzheimer's disease.

- People with schizophrenia have fewer and more poorly functioning nicotinic receptors. Up to 80% of people with schizophrenia smoke (and they inhale more deeply), and they likely experience improvement in their cognitive, sensory, social, and emotional experience. Research is being conducted on nicotine as a potential medication.

- More teens who suffer from depression smoke, which may be an attempt to medicate this disorder.

Risks and Harmful Effects

Dependence, Tolerance, and Withdrawal

Tolerance develops to both the physical and mental effects of nicotine. The first cigarette after a period of abstinence is the most potent and can cause dizziness, nausea, and sometimes vomiting. Since nicotine stimulates dopamine, it is reinforcing and therefore has great addictive potential. Withdrawal consists of extreme cravings and irritability for at least 2 to 3 weeks. Occasionally people report nausea and vomiting in withdrawal. Many people who have successfully quit other drugs report that they have the hardest time giving up cigarettes.

Medical Risks

Although at high doses nicotine is highly toxic, most of the harms of nicotine are due to the delivery system. Tobacco is the psychoactive drug responsible for more deaths in the United States than all other drugs, including alcohol: 480,000 in 2014, including 40,000 from passive smoke.

- Ingestion of carbon monoxide and tar deprives the body of oxygen and sticks to the fibers in the lungs. The combination of carbon monoxide and oxygen deprivation may counteract the potential good effects on attention and memory.

- Smoking causes various lung diseases (chronic obstructive pulmonary disease, chronic bronchitis, emphysema) and cancers of the lungs, mouth, throat.

- Cardiovascular damage: increased heart rate leads to the need for increased oxygen supply, which is depleted and replaced with carbon monoxide. This depletion causes stress and damage to the heart. Arteriosclerosis, hardening of the arteries, and atherosclerosis, the buildup of fatty deposits in the arteries, are associated with smoking. Up to 30% of cardiovascular deaths are due to smoking.

- Thinning of the skin as smokers age, possibly due to oxygen deprivation.

- Nicotine passes through the blood–placenta barrier, causing lower birth weight in babies and possible learning deficits.

- Children of men who smoke are at increased risk of getting cancer, possibly due to damaged sperm and altered DNA.

Practicing Harm Reduction

Quitting seems to be the best way of reducing harm, since the drug is so reinforcing that controlling use can be difficult, although there are plenty of occasional or casual smokers. The chances of quitting are vastly better if one uses two or more interventions—medication, counseling, and/or peer support.

If you don't quit:

- *Try e-cigarettes!* Despite the media frenzy, most of the available research shows that vaporizing tobacco reduces the health hazards by up to 95%. Even though these products are enormously safer than cigarettes, nicotine is still easy to get hooked on, so it's not a great idea to start using e-cigs if you are not already dependent on nicotine. (Recent research indicates that added flavorings in e-cigs can cause lung conditions that are often disabling or fatal.)

- Don't smoke where you can affect others.

- Avoid using at times when you don't really need or want a cigarette (don't use automatically).

- Decide on a certain number of cigarettes a day (such as five or eight) and smoke only that much.

- Don't smoke at all one or more days a week.

- Switch to a lower tar and nicotine brand.

- Use a nicotine patch or gum in place of some of your cigarettes (be careful, though; too much can make you sick).

- Manipulate your environment: spend more time in places where you can't smoke.

- Don't smoke cigarettes while pregnant. E-cigarettes will reduce harm.

- Limit your smoking while trying to become pregnant (women *and* men).

Medication-Assisted Treatment

- Zyban (bupropion, an antidepressant medication) can help to reduce cravings for up to 12 weeks.

- Nicotine patches administer nicotine through your skin and help reduce your reliance on cigarettes.

- Chantix, a nonnicotine medication, targets the nicotinic receptors so that your brain "thinks" it is smoking.

Caffeine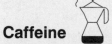

Found in **coffee, tea, soft drinks, "energy" drinks, chocolate, kola (or cola) nuts, over-the-counter pain relievers, performance drugs,** and **prescription medications.**

Caffeine is the most widely used drug in the world. It belongs to a class of stimulant drugs called *xanthines,* a family that includes caffeine, theophylline, which is found in tea, and theobromine, found in chocolate. Tea, the world's oldest caffeine-containing beverage, can be traced back to 2700 B.C. in China, where it was thought to have medicinal properties. It was introduced to Europe by the Dutch in the early 1600s, though it was the British and Russians who adopted it as a national drink. Coffee, called "the wine of Islam," originated in Ethiopia. Colas are made from the African cola nut, which is very bitter and is chewed for its stimulating effect. Little cola is left in sodas, but it is one of the original ingredients, along with extract of cocaine, of the original Coca-Cola. Guarana, the national drink of Brazil, made from the seeds of a bush, contains more caffeine than coffee and is made into sodas. Mate, the national drink of Argentina, sometimes sold as an herbal tea in the United States, does contain caffeine.

The amount of caffeine in different substances (in milligrams) varies widely and is always listed on the packaging. The differences among energy drinks, for example, can be significant.

How It Works

Caffeine's main action is to block adenosine, which sedates brain activity. Two cups of coffee stimulate brain activity. Caffeine increases adrenaline, which heightens alertness, euphoria, heart rate, and blood pressure. Caffeine causes the kidneys to release urine. It increases urinary excretion of calcium and slows absorption of calcium. It relaxes the smooth muscles in the bronchioles and can ease breathing. It also constricts blood vessels, which is useful for treating headaches and is often an ingredient in headache medicines.

For unknown reasons, the effects of coffee and pure caffeine differ—coffee seems to be more potent than pure caffeine or other caffeine-containing plants.

Flavonoids, compounds that act as antioxidants in the blood and prevent the development of arteriosclerosis and atherosclerosis, are found in cocoa. Three table-spoons of cocoa powder or a 1.5-ounce piece of chocolate contains approximately the same amount of flavonoids as a 5-ounce glass of red wine. But milk chocolate contains milk fat and other saturated fats that can negate this positive effect.

Beneficial Effects

- Energy, alertness, and concentration. Caffeine serves as a milder stimulant than amphetamines, and it's cheaper and legal!

- Improves reaction time and coordination and is an overall performance enhancer.

- Headache remedy.

- Improves speed and endurance.

- Many social benefits.

Risks and Harmful Effects

Dependence, Tolerance, and Withdrawal

People become dependent on coffee and other caffeinated beverages quickly. Tolerance to and dependence on coffee is common in Western societies. Withdrawal symptoms begin about 24 hours after the last dose and include a vascular headache that can be severe, irritability, nausea, and lethargy. Withdrawal tends to last up to 3 days.

- Increased bone loss in postmenopausal women at levels of three cups of coffee or five cups of tea a day (due to caffeine's effect on calcium elimination and absorption).

- Anxiety and insomnia. Consumption of four to five cups of coffee a day can precipitate a panic attack in those with a history of anxiety or panic.

- Nervousness and tremulousness at high doses.

- Increases high blood pressure.

- Diuretic at higher doses (three to five cups of coffee, five to eight cups of tea), contributing to dehydration.

- Some studies report low birth weight for babies of coffee drinkers. At the end of pregnancy or while taking oral contraceptives, caffeine is eliminated more slowly, and a buildup can occur that causes symptoms of caffeine intoxication.

- Restricts blood flow in the eyes, decreasing nutrients and clearing of waste.

- Caffeine is generally not dangerous; however, 800 milligrams of caffeine could be toxic in a small child (about eight cups of coffee or 2 pounds of chocolate). Toxic symptoms are upset stomach, vomiting, extreme nervousness, and nervous system stimulation, which could lead to seizures.

Note to parents of young children: The effects of caffeine listed above reflect adult doses. These effects will be compounded in children, as the last example shows.

Practicing Harm Reduction

Since caffeine products are legal and pleasing to many, a general harm reduction advisory should suffice. The poison is in the dose, and the risks depend on the person and the situation. Don't be fooled by decaf—it contains small amounts of caffeine and all of the other irritants to the gastrointestinal, cardiovascular, and urinary systems. If you suffer from anxiety, nervousness, trouble sleeping, heart palpitations, or upset stomach, try cutting back or eliminating caffeine as a first experiment. You'll be surprised by how much it helps. If you want lower doses of caffeine in your coffee, arabica has less caffeine than cheaper robusta, as do darker roasts.

Hallucinogens/Psychedelics

There are many hallucinogens and many excellent sources of information about them. Each group works in a different way. Here we list many of them and address as much as we can in our limited space. For more information on each drug, the Vaults of Erowid website (*www.erowid.org*) is a good place to go, as is the book *Buzzed* (Kuhn, Swartzwelder, and Wilson).

- *Serotonin-related* (chemically similar to serotonin): **LSD,** synthetically derived from ergot, a fungus in moldy rye; **Ololiuqui** (morning-glory seeds); **psilocybin** (mushrooms); **DMT** (dimethyltryptamine), found in the bark of some trees and nuts in Central and South America; **harmine,** found in the bark of a South American vine; **bufotenine,** found in the venom of certain toads.

- *Catecholamine-related* (similar to norepinephrine): **mescaline,** the active ingredient in the peyote cactus in Mexico and the U.S. Southwest; **DOM** or **STP,** a synthetic mescaline-like compound, not much used because it is very potent—dosages are not well controlled, and toxic reactions are common.

- *Acetylcholine-related* (similar to acetylcholine): **atropine** and **scopolamine,** found in belladonna or deadly nightshade and datura plants (including jimsonweed); **ibogaine** (ibotenic acid), found in *Amanita mascaria* mushrooms and the iboga plant.

- *Opioid kappa-receptor agonists*: **Salvia divinorum,** the only form of the salvia plant family that has hallucinogenic properties. It has been used in religious rituals in Mexico for centuries.

The term *hallucinogenic* refers to the ability of a drug or substance to produce hallucinations, which are perceptions of visions, sounds, or smells that are not real. Hallucinogenic drugs more often intensify or alter perceptions rather than creating ones that are not there. However, the power is in the dose. At very high doses, these drugs can actually produce true hallucinations. The most popularized term for this type of experience is *psychedelic,* referring to the drugs' positive abilities to create "mind-expanding" experiences.

Some of these compounds are the products of plants found in different parts of the world and have been in cultural or religious use for hundreds or thousands of years. The synthetic compounds were all developed in the 20th century for a variety of reasons, often unrelated to their current recreational use.

Actions and Effects

In general, these drugs either stimulate or suppress the activity of the neurotransmitter most similar to them. The serotonin-related drugs and the norepinephrine-related drugs tend to *stimulate* some of the receptors that cause hallucinations when not in balance with the others. The acetylcholine-related drugs *block* acetylcholine, which slows the heart and helps to form memories. When used respectfully and in the right circumstances, these drugs give a sense of expansiveness and connectedness as well as visions or insights that would otherwise be unattainable. Some people use them in friendship groups to enhance social interactions and fun. Others use them in a more ritualized way to expand consciousness and aid in their spiritual development.

Serotonin-Related Hallucinogens

Effects vary depending on which drug is used, the person's expectations, and the setting. Hallucinogens are among the most set- and setting-dependent of drugs. Mild effects include detachment and an altered sense of space and time. Higher doses cause visual disturbances and hallucinations, depersonalization, intense feelings of insight, a sense of being very focused, and synesthesia (confusion of senses— "hearing sights" or "seeing sounds"). They do not cause a real psychotic experience, but they can trigger psychosis in a vulnerable person. DMT, from Central and South America, is a short-acting hallucinogen, causing a trip of just an hour—the "businessman's lunch." It is so quick, it is more likely to cause anxiety. DMT is metabolized by monoamine oxidase (MAO).

Catecholamine-Related Hallucinogens

Physical effects are similar to those produced by amphetamine. Psychological effects are similar to those experienced on LSD, and a trip can last from 30 minutes to over 12 hours, depending on the drug. Nausea is a common initial effect of these substances.

One example in this class is peyote. Peyote has been used for at least 3,000 years in Mexico (including what is now the U.S. Southwest). It was used by the Mescalero Apaches in the 19th century, thus the name of the active ingredient *mescaline*. Peyote was officially incorporated into the Native American Church of North America in the early 20th century and is used as a sacrament. The cactus buttons are sliced, dried, and then eaten. Otherwise, a tea is made from them.

Acetylcholine-Related Hallucinogens

Atropine and scopolamine are usually the active ingredients. Atropine can give the feeling of flying, possibly contributing to the idea from the Middle Ages that witches can fly. It causes a bizarre dreamlike state and increased heart rate and temperature. It is a bronchodilator and causes amnesia.

Belladonna, or deadly nightshade, has historically been used as a poison, as a medicine to treat asthma, as a beauty aid (it dilates the pupils, considered appealing in women), and ritually for thousands of years. Recreational use is recent.

Datura, or jimsonweed, causes a hypnotic, hallucinogenic experience, as well as disorientation, confusion, and amnesia. It is toxic at high doses.

Ibogaine is derived from the iboga root in Africa and has been used in tribal ceremonies in Gabon and the Congo as an aid in seeking advice from ancestors.

The root is chewed, and intoxication can last for 30 hours. Ibogaine is now used as a therapeutic drug to help reduce cocaine, alcohol, nicotine, and opioid dependence.

Risks and Harmful Effects

Dependence, Tolerance, and Withdrawal

Users develop a tolerance to the effects of some of these drugs, but since there is little to no stimulation of dopamine, there is low dependence potential and no withdrawal.

- Accidents and physical injury have been reported during bad trips or due to disorientation from some drugs.

- Anxiety and nausea are not uncommon with high doses (sometimes nausea is a normal part of the experience).

- Flashbacks may be related to memory changes. There is some evidence that the brain responds to stimuli and recalls stored memories. Up to 60% of heavy users experience flashbacks; they are not usually perceived as scary or dangerous.

- Underlying psychosis can be triggered by use of hallucinogens.

Practicing Harm Reduction

- Plan your trip—it's most enjoyable then—and allow plenty of time. You'll probably be tired the next day.

- Know your dose.

- Use with people you know and with whom you feel safe. Keep an eye on each other.

- Use one drug at a time.

- Be careful with all of the acetylcholine-related drugs. **These can be lethal at doses that are not much higher than the recreational dose.**

- Don't pick mushrooms unless you are experienced.

- A full stomach will increase the likelihood of getting nauseous, so eat just a little, if at all.

- Anxiety can be treated with reassurance or benzodiazepines.

- Do not drive or try to operate other machinery.

Ecstasy (MDMA)

MDMA (ecstasy) and **MDA** are synthetic compounds and also considered entacto-gens ("touch within") or empathogens, not strictly hallucinogenic. MDMA belongs to both the hallucinogen and the stimulant classes of drugs. Developed in the 1930s as an experimental amphetamine to be used as a compound in other drugs, MDMA was never used, nor was it studied. It was revived in the 1980s for use as an empathy enhancer in couple therapy. According to the federal government, it was toxic and had no proven medical effect, so it was placed on the Schedule I list. But it does not, in fact, seem to be toxic with occasional use, which is how many, if not most, people use it. Ecstasy is currently being researched as a treatment for PTSD.

How It Works

Ecstasy increases levels of serotonin, which creates feelings of well-being. Ecstasy floods the synapses with serotonin, which explains its dramatic effect on mood. As an "excitatory" neurotransmitter, it also causes the release of dopamine and norepinephrine. Ecstasy is usually taken in pill form—50–150 milligrams—and is sometimes cut with caffeine, ephedrine, or dextromethorphan. Its effects peak in 1 hour and can last 3–6 hours. It is considered to have the stimulant effects of amphetamines and the hallucinogenic qualities of mescaline. As an amphetamine-based drug, it increases heart rate, blood pressure, and body temperature; dilates bronchioles and pupils; increases blood flow to muscles; and lowers appetite. It does not cause real hallucinations, but time perception is distorted.

Beneficial Effects

The experience of warmth, empathy, and closeness with others is viewed as one of the primary benefits of using these drugs. In addition, it is sometimes used for "journeys of the soul" or to help resolve emotional issues.

- Sense of empathy and openness.
- Lowers fear and defensiveness and decreases one's sense of separateness, aggression, and obsessiveness.
- Can stimulate sexual interest as an offshoot of the sense of openness, although serotonin itself can actually decrease sexual drive.
- When taken at parties or dance clubs, the stimulant qualities provide energy and a sense of excitement and euphoria.
- Research into MDMA as a treatment for PTSD is very promising.

Risks and Harmful Effects

Dependence, Tolerance, and Withdrawal

Ecstasy is generally used in specific circumstances and not in a typically addictive pattern of compulsive use. In fact, overuse is difficult, since tolerance develops rapidly and it depletes the brain's store of serotonin molecules and "down-regulates" the serotonin receptors, thus making it impossible to get "high" after a few doses. MDMA does not appear to cause dependence, nor a true withdrawal, but after-effects of intoxication often result in the experience of depression, since serotonin neurotransmitters are exhausted. It takes 10–14 days to regenerate one's supply of serotonin.

Medical Risks

- Ecstasy is often cut with other substances, commonly "bath salts," stimulants, ketamine, or dextromethorphan. One test of a sample of ecstasy pills showed that only 40% of them contained just ecstasy. The rest contained either a little ecstasy or none at all. For the occasional or regular (but not heavy) user, ecstasy is not particularly toxic. The problem is that, since there is so little pure ecstasy, you can easily get toxic reactions such as agitation, paranoia, or hallucinations, which are not typical reactions to ecstasy.

- Ecstasy raises body temperature at high doses (only two to three times a single dose), which causes dehydration, muscle breakdown, and kidney failure. As a result, some people have died of hyperthermia. Increasing doses produce symptoms of jitteriness, teeth clenching, cramping, nausea, paranoia, dizziness, crankiness, weakness, and lack of coordination.

- As the dose increases, so do the negative effects on the brain. Large doses taken at once can eliminate the ability of the serotonin system to work for weeks afterward, resulting in mood disorders and memory problems. Heavy use (100 times over a few years) can cause significant neurotoxicity, mostly by disabling the serotonin system as well as creating long-standing memory deficits. While ecstasy impairs memory during intoxication, unless one is a heavy user, it does not seem to have any long-standing negative effects on memory or other cognitive functions.

Drug Interactions

- MAO inhibitors (MAOIs, one type of antidepressant medication) increase the supply of serotonin and, in conjunction with ecstasy, increase the likelihood of serotonin syndrome, a potentially fatal condition characterized by increased body temperature, muscle rigidity, and high fever.

- Any drugs that increase heart rate, blood pressure, temperature, or dehydration—stimulants, alcohol, or dextromethorphan, for example—have a greater risk of these symptoms when combined with ecstasy.

- Alcohol increases the dehydrating effects of ecstasy.

Practicing Harm Reduction

- If you can, test your pills for purity. There are labs in the United States that can test, but you have to send in a sample, which takes time, so plan ahead! Dance-Safe, a harm reduction organization, used to work at some clubs and raves, where workers offered pill-testing kits. They are no longer allowed access, but they have a lot of good information about safety on their website and an online store where you can buy personal drug-testing kits.

- Drink *water,* not alcohol, when using ecstasy. Don't go overboard—it doesn't take a lot of water to stay hydrated, and too much can upset the delicate balance of electrolytes.

- Stay cool—wear cool clothes and avoid headgear; dab the back of your neck and your wrists with cool water.

- **Call 911 if you see anyone showing signs of hyperthermia, confusion, nausea, or unconsciousness.**

Designer Drugs

People synthesize new drugs every day, so the list is endless. Often the goal is to create drugs with effects that are similar to those of drugs that have been banned. Here is a list of the most common current ones:

- 2CB, DOM

- Bath salts (mephedrone and MDPV)

- Spice (synthetic cannabis), or K2

- Other synthetic "hallucinogens": AMT and 5-MeO-DIPT (Foxy), BZP and TFMPP, 2C-I-NBOMe (Smiles, N-Bomb)

How They Work and Why They Are Used

Many of these drugs are used widely as party drugs. Others are experimental in that people manipulate the chemical composition of a drug to see what other effects can be achieved. The experience of warmth, empathy, and closeness with others is viewed as one of the primary benefits of using many of these drugs. When taken at parties or dance clubs, the stimulant qualities provide energy and a sense of excitement and euphoria. And many people increase the dose precisely because they are looking for a new hallucinogenic experience. At higher doses, the "out of body, out of mind" loss of control is extremely pleasant for some people and not for others.

The drugs *2CB* and *DOM* are both analogues of mescaline. They have the effect at lower doses of making people feel "in touch" with themselves. At higher doses, they produce vivid hallucinations but with more mental clarity than other hallucinogens. They are usually taken orally in tablets or gel caps. More like ecstasy than a hallucinogen, 2CB is considered an entactogen. DOM is very dose sensitive, with little margin between toxic and recreational doses, and it is difficult to know the dose in a tablet. There have been some reports of nausea, chills, trembling, and convulsive movements. How it actually works is unknown.

Bath salts are synthetic, nonamphetamine stimulants that belong in the synthetic cathinone category (khat is a natural cathinone). Mephedrone is usually the main ingredient, and it is also related to MDMA, although its effects are more erratic. Another ingredient of bath salts is often MDPV. People react very differently to these products, perhaps because the products themselves are not consistent in terms of what is in them or the dose, and partly because each person may have his or her own idiosyncratic reaction. Many people feel a mild euphoria and stimulation, while a certain minority of people become agitated, paranoid, and have panic attacks. Extreme states of psychosis and paranoia can occur.

Spice (herbal/synthetic cannabis) consists of plant material that has been sprayed or soaked with several different hallucinogenic compounds that mimic THC, such as XLR-11. This drug can be a mild intoxicant or can be soaked with large amounts of other drugs, so it is difficult to tell with each batch not only how strong it is but also whether the mixers are something that you will not like. People report feeling paranoid, "out of it," or sick to their stomach. Users have had severe reactions to some batches that caused incoordination, seizures, catatonia, and nausea and vomiting.

AMT and *5-MeO-DIPT (Foxy)* are both synthetic hallucinogens, with AMT having a slow onset and longer activity and Foxy coming on rapidly and lasting only 3–6 hours. Foxy can cause significant confusion, so it's best to use with others who may not have taken it.

BZP and *TFMPP* belong to the piperazine class of drugs and are often combined in the same "party pill." Low doses cause stimulation and euphoria, but at higher doses hallucinogenic and toxic effects predominate. Headache, vomiting, seizures, and organ damage can occur at higher doses.

Sometimes sold as "Super-Ecstasy," *2C-I (Smiles, N-Bomb)* is a fairly recent designer drug and not available in many places. Similar to DOM, it causes euphoria at lower doses and agitation, confusion, and hallucinations at higher ones.

Risks and Harmful Effects

The biggest risk with designer drugs is not knowing where they were manufactured or by whom. Many of the pills and/or ingredients of bath salts and Spice are manufactured in China or India. Of course, quality control of illicit substance manufacture is nonexistent. Some drugs may be made in household settings, some with good chemistry technique and some not.

Dependence, Tolerance, and Withdrawal

None of these drugs are known for dependence, tolerance, or withdrawal, which does not mean that it isn't possible. Their use as experimental or party drugs tends to mitigate against regular use that could lead to dependence.

Practicing Harm Reduction

Just Say Know. In the case of designer drugs it's really *know thy chemist* and *know thy dose*. Many of these drugs offer perfectly safe recreation at low doses, but at higher doses or in combination can result in some pretty nasty trips as well as organ damage.

Dissociative Anesthetics

Ketamine, phencyclidine (PCP), dextromethorphan (DXM), nitrous oxide (laughing gas): These drugs are sometimes classified as hallucinogens or psychedelics, but their physical effects are so different from those of the other hallucinogens, and there are such specific risk factors associated with their use, that we have separated them here. They all block the action of NMDA glutamate receptors in the brain, which results in slowed thinking and reactions.

Both ketamine and PCP (angel dust) were developed as surgical anesthetics that had the advantage of not depressing respiration or blood pressure or causing heart irregularities. But they had a tendency to cause psychiatric symptoms similar to those of schizophrenia, causing them to be restricted primarily to use in veterinary medicine. They are still used in human medicine where respiratory depression is a concern during surgery.

PCP's effects look like a combination of those of alcohol, amphetamines, and hallucinogens. Signs of PCP intoxication include slurred speech; impaired coordination; increased heart rate, blood pressure, and temperature; a dissociative state; and lowered sensitivity to pain and occasionally increased belligerence.

Ketamine has been used as a club drug in both the gay and straight party scenes since the 1980s. It is also used by people who want a spiritual experience. Ketamine can be taken orally, snorted, or injected intravenously or intramuscularly. It can also cause hallucinations, disorientation, delayed nightmares, dizziness, confusion, slurred speech, and amnesia. Ketamine dramatically lowers one's ability to move or feel pain. Most recently, ketamine has been studied as a new class of antidepressant medication for people who have treatment-resistant depression.

Dextromethorphan (DXM) is a nonopioid cough suppressant in several over-the-counter cough syrups. It prevents the reuptake of dopamine and stimulates heart rate, blood pressure, and sweating. It takes at least 4 ounces to get high, and the high can last 10 hours.

Nitrous oxide was developed in 1798 by a British chemist who noticed a very pleasant effect of lightness and giddiness. Nicknamed "laughing gas," it was used recreationally at parties as a nonalcoholic intoxicant in Britain and the United States. In the 1840s, a dentist using it recreationally noticed that people felt no pain while high. He started using it in his dental practice. Nitrous creates feelings of euphoria, behavioral disinhibition, and pain reduction for a few minutes, as well as a feeling of well-being for several hours. Occasional loss of consciousness is followed by sensory distortion and nausea. When used recreationally, it is dispensed from tanks diverted from medical usage and then used to fill balloons to breathe from, or in the form of "whippets," the gas delivery system in cans of whipped cream. Nitrous can also be classified as an inhalant.

Beneficial Effects

Dissociative anesthetics dissolve self-consciousness, create a sense of detachment, increase tolerance for physical pain, and decrease fear and anxiety. The "K-hole," the ultimate ketamine experience, is a dreamlike state in which people report feeling one with the universe and at peace. This is the experience that some users seek. Others find the experience terrifying.

Risks and Harmful Effects

Dependence, Tolerance, and Withdrawal

In general, tolerance does not develop to these drugs, and if it does, it tends to occur gradually over time with repeated doses. They do not tend to cause either dependence or withdrawal, although some people say that they experience cravings.

Medical Risks

- PCP can cause psychosis, accidents, and fights. At high doses, it can cause general anesthesia, very high temperature, increased blood pressure (which can cause stroke), seizure, coma, decreased respiration, a psychotic state, extreme agitation, belligerence, and traumatic injury. It is an unpredictable drug that may be added to other drugs, so be careful.

- People on ketamine can fall if they try to move around; they may also experience nausea and vomiting, breathing problems, racing heart, and confusion. Ketamine can cause psychosis in vulnerable people.

- Nitrous is very cold and can damage the lungs, cause accidents when movement is attempted, and deplete the body of vitamin B_{12}, which can lead to neuropathy (damage to the peripheral nerves) over time; damage also can be caused by expanding gas overinflating the lungs, trachea, or mouth. It deprives the brain and body of oxygen in proportion to how much is breathed. Nitrous can cause suffocation due to carbon dioxide buildup, especially when the nitrous in a balloon is recycled.

- Cough syrups containing DXM can cause nausea and an extremely elevated temperature.

- All dissociative anesthetics have some potential for causing brain damage, although the research is quite contradictory. It is possible that the longer you use, and the higher the doses you take, the greater the risk.

Drug Interactions

- Any drugs that lower the seizure threshold (for example, the antidepressant Wellbutrin, GHB, stimulants) increase the risk of seizure because the brain is already stimulated.

- Any drugs that decrease respiration increase the risk of overdose, with coma being the most dangerous point.

- Ritalin and ketamine may create a condition called *chemical hepatitis*. Stimulants further increase blood pressure and heart rate and cause risk of stroke.

- Marijuana at high doses may increase the dissociative experience.

- Other hallucinogens may tend to make the drug experience too intense.

Practicing Harm Reduction

- Use as little as possible of these drugs. Try to limit your use to no more than two times a week and space the use so that you have a couple of days in between.

- Take extra vitamin B_{12} if you use nitrous.

- Do not drive or operate other machinery. Watch out for your friends and yourself. Use somewhere that is safe and comfortable.

- If you are responsible for someone's care (child, elder, or person with serious illness), avoid using these drugs at that time. It's just too hard to pull it together when on these drugs.

- We need a mix of at least 21% oxygen in the air we breathe. It is important to breathe in between doses of nitrous. Do not breathe directly from a tank! The pressure can tear your lung tissue. Do not recirculate nitrous in the balloon; doing so causes a buildup of carbon dioxide.

Deliriants/Inhalants

Nitrites: butyl or amyl nitrite (poppers); **solvents (paint thinners and removers) and cleaning solutions:** contain carbon tetrachloride, petroleum products, and trichloroethylene; **glues, paints, spray paints:** contain acetone, butylacetate methanol, and toluene; **sprays** (such as hair spray, deodorants, and air fresheners): contain butane and propane; **nail polish remover:** contains acetone; **lighter fluids:** contain butane and isopropane; **fuels** such as gasoline: contain petroleum products.

Nitrites have been used for medical purposes since the mid–19th century. They have the same effects as nitroglycerin (discovered in 1846), an explosive also used to dilate blood vessels in heart patients when the heart spasms.

Solvents are not intended for human consumption. They are volatile compounds developed for household and industrial use as cleaners and solvents. Because they are cheap or free and easily available, they are used by the youngest of drug users, particularly in poor areas. Of all psychoactive substances, they are the most destructive in that they routinely cause brain, lung, and liver damage. They have effects similar to those of alcohol and anesthetics: euphoria and initial stimulation, followed by central nervous system depression. In addition, routine use depresses the immune system, and the lack of coordination can lead to devastating falls.

Beneficial Effects

- Alterations in consciousness

- Reduced ability to feel pain, loss of muscle control

- Euphoria leading to dissociative states

As with all psychoactive substances, the ability of inhalants to alter experience and get one "out of it" is attractive and often fun. In the case of solvents, this is all that can be said of their benefits. Nitrites are more specific in their recreational effects, particularly with regard to enhancing sexual pleasure and creating feelings of well-being and stimulation.

Nitrites relax smooth muscle tissue, which regulates the size of blood vessels, the bladder, and the anus (thereby facilitating anal sex). They both lower blood pressure and increase heart rate, and create a sense of warmth, lowered inhibition, euphoria, exhilaration, and acceleration before orgasm.

Risks and Harmful Effects

Dependence, Tolerance, and Withdrawal

Tolerance develops to nitrites, and cardiac problems can occur in withdrawal as the blood vessels contract in the absence of the drug. The same symptoms appear as when one started using—headaches, dizziness, and weakness.

Medical Risks

Nitrites

- Headaches, dizziness, and loss of consciousness if one tries to move rapidly.

- If swallowed, they prevent blood from transporting oxygen, which can lead to death.

- Immune suppression, but as is the case for many illegal substances, very little solid research has been done.

- Poppers also may suppress the immune system for several days after use. They are not recommended for people with low or high blood pressure.

Solvents

- Incoordination, hallucinations, delusions, flushing, double vision, suppression of vital functions like respiration and heart function, and impaired judgment.

- Other than brief intoxication, these chemicals cause nothing but damage, especially to the cerebellum, which controls fine-motor skills.

- Memory, attention, and concentration are affected, and two studies found that 55–65% of patients admitted to emergency rooms after sniffing solvents suffered central nervous system damage.

- Because of the intense disorientation and incoordination, 26% of deaths from inhalants are from accidents. Another 28% of deaths are by suicide. Many of those who die are first-time users.

- "Sudden sniffing death," likely due to interrupting the heart rhythm and increasing its sensitivity to adrenaline, can occur when sniffing gaseous substances such as freon, butane, or propane.

Drug Interactions

- When using these inhalants, the most important drugs to avoid using simultaneously are central nervous system depressants such as alcohol, sedatives, or opioids.

- Using nitrous and ketamine together might increase neurotoxicity.

- Do not mix poppers with Viagra—the interaction may lead to dangerously low blood pressure.

Practicing Harm Reduction

It is tempting to say "Just Say No" to solvents. Since, as harm reductionists, we can't just tell you what to do and expect that you'll do it—and at least 20% of U.S. and European high school kids have tried solvents, and millions of children in Latin America, South Asia, and Africa use them—we recommend that you at least try to minimize some of the risk:

- Use as little and as seldom as possible. Plan your use, enjoy it while it lasts, but put your heart through these changes as little as possible. **Call 911 if you swallow poppers.**

- Remember that other drugs can get you high and do far less damage than these.

- Move around as little as possible to avoid accidents.

- If you feel suicidal, get your friend(s) to help you find someone you can trust to talk to.

- Don't drive or operate other machinery.

- As with any drug that causes disorientation, if you are a parent or a caretaker, plan your use for times when you don't have to take care of anyone.

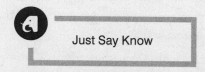

Just Say Know

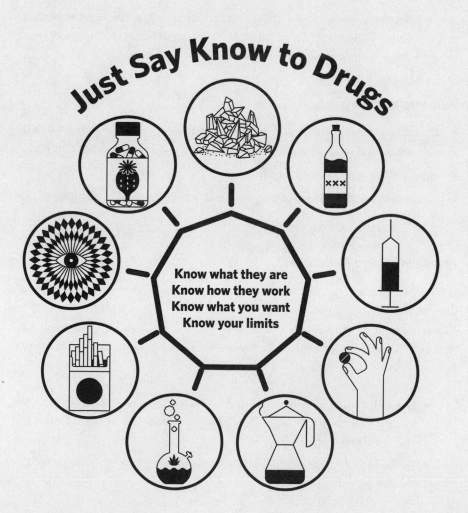

Resources

Harm Reduction–Oriented Substance Use Treatment, Self-Help Programs, and Other Resources

Please note: The following are well-established organizations led by seasoned substance use treatment professionals, but there are others not listed, including many individual harm reduction therapy practitioners. If you contact us, we will do our best to connect you with treatment resources in your area.

Licensed and/or Certified Substance Use and Mental Health Treatment Programs

The Center for Harm Reduction Therapy
Patt Denning, PhD, and Jeannie Little, LCSW
San Francisco, Oakland, San Jose, and Mill Valley, CA
      Therapists also available at Homeless Youth Alliance, Hospitality House, San Francisco AIDS Foundation's Harm Reduction Center, San Francisco LGBT Center Youth Program, and San Mateo County HIV Programs
415-863-4282
www.harmreductiontherapy.org

The Center for Optimal Living
Andrew Tatarsky, PhD
New York, NY
212-213-8905
www.harmreductioncounseling.com

Center for Motivation and Change
Jeff Foote, PhD, and Carrie Wilkins, PhD
New York and Massachusetts
212-683-3339; 413-229-3333
www.motivationandchange.com

Practical Recovery
A. Thomas Horvath, PhD
La Jolla, CA
800-977-6110
www.practicalrecovery.com

Addiction Alternatives
Marc Kern, PhD, and Adi Jaffe, PhD
Los Angeles, CA
888-532-9137, ext. 102
www.habitdoc.com
www.addictionalternatives.com

**Healthy Lifestyles Guided Self-Change Program,
Nova Southeastern University**
Linda Sobell, PhD, and Mark Sobell, PhD
Fort Lauderdale, FL
800-541-6682, ext. 25968
www.nova.edu/gsc

The Stonewall Project
San Francisco AIDS Foundation
www.stonewallsf.org

Minnesota Alternatives
Paula DeSanto MS, LSW, CPRP, CCDP-D
7766 NE Hwy. 65
Spring Lake Park, MN 55432
and
1650 Carroll Ave.
St Paul, MN 55104
763-789-4895
www.mnalternatives.com

Self-Help Groups and Online Programs

CheckUp and Choices, *www.checkupandchoices.com*

HAMS (Harm Reduction, Abstinence, and Moderation Support),
www.hamsnetwork.org

LifeRing Secular Recovery, *www.lifering.org*

Moderation Management, *www.moderation.org*

Refuge Recovery, *www.refugerecovery.org*

Secular Organizations for Sobriety (SOS),
www.cfiwest.org/sos www.centerforinquiry.net

SMART Recovery, *www.smartrecovery.org*

St. James Infirmary, *www.stjamesinfirmary.org* (information for sex workers)

Women for Sobriety (WFS), *www.womenforsobriety.org*

Public Health Harm Reduction Programs (many include counseling)

Fortunately, there are now many harm reduction organizations around the world. Below we highlight national and regional harm reduction coalitions (this is not a complete list!) and the Drug Policy Alliance, which list harm reduction organizations on their websites. And of course you can do a web search for syringe exchange, drug user health, or harm reduction.

Atlanta Harm Reduction Coalition, *www.atlantaharmreduction.org*

Canadian Harm Reduction Network, *www.canadianharmreduction.com*

The Chicago Recovery Alliance (CRA), *www.anypositivechange.org*

DanceSafe (Drug information and pill testing), *www.dancesafe.org*

Drug Policy Alliance, *www.drugpolicy.org*

Harm Reduction Action Center (Denver), *www.harmreductionactioncenter.org*

Harm Reduction Australia, *www.harmreductionaustralia.org.au*

Harm Reduction Coalition, *www.harmreduction.org*

Insite Vancouver Coastal Health Supervised Injection Site, *www.vch.ca/public-health/harm-reduction/supervised-injection-sites*

The Irish Needle Exchange Forum, *www.inef.ie*

North American Syringe Exchange Network, *www.nasen.org*

North Carolina Harm Reduction Coalition, *www.nchrc.org*

Syringe Access Program, San Francisco AIDS Foundation, *www.sfaf.org/client-services/syringe-access*

UK Harm Reduction Alliance, *www.ukhra.org*

Books, Pamphlets, and Online Resources

AA—Not the Only Way: Your One Stop Resource Guide to 12-Step Alternatives. Melanie Solomon. *www.aanottheonlyway.com*.

Addiction and Change: How Addictions Develop and Addicted People Recover. Carlo DiClemente. Guilford Press. 2006.

Changing for Good: The Revolutionary Program That Explains the Six Stages of Change and Teaches You How to Free Yourself from Bad Habits. James Prochaska, John Norcross, and Carlo DiClemente. Avon Books. 1994.

Controlling Your Drinking: Tools to Make Moderation Work for You (2nd ed.). William Miller and Ricardo Munoz. Guilford Press. 2013.

Finding Your Way to Change: How the Power of Motivational Interviewing Can Reveal What You Want and Help You Get There. Allan Zuckoff. Guilford Press. 2015.

Getting Off Right: A Safety Manual for Injection Drug Users. Rod Sorge and Sara Kershnar. Harm Reduction Coalition. 1998. PDF available at *www.harmreduction. org/drugs-and-drug-users/drug-tools/getting-off-right*.

Her Best-Kept Secret: Why Women Drink—And How They Can Regain Control. Gabrielle Glaser. Simon & Schuster. 2013.

How to Change Your Drinking: A Harm Reduction Guide to Alcohol (2nd ed.). Kenneth Anderson. HAMS Harm Reduction Network. 2010.

Recovery Options: The Complete Guide. Joseph Volpicelli and Maia Szalavitz. Wiley. 2000.

Resisting 12-Step Coercion: How to Fight Forced Participation in AA, NA, or 12-Step Treatment. Stanton Peele, Charles Bufe, and Archie Brodsky. See Sharp Press. 2000.

Responsible Drinking: A Moderation Management Approach for Problem Drinkers. Frederick Rotgers, Marc Kern, and Rudy Hoeltzel. New Harbinger. 2002.

Rethinking Drinking: Alcohol and Your Health. National Institute on Alcohol Abuse and Alcoholism. *http://pubs.niaaa.nih.gov/publications/RethinkingDrinking/OrderPage.htm.*

Sex, Drugs, Gambling, and Chocolate: A Workbook for Overcoming Addictions. A. Thomas Horvath. Impact. 1998.

Sober for Good: New Solutions for Drinking Problems—Advice from Those Who Have Succeeded. Anne Fletcher. Houghton Mifflin. 2002.

Drug Information

The Botany of Desire: A Plant's-Eye View of the World. Michael Pollan. Random House. 2001. (See the chapter on marijuana.)

Buzzed: The Straight Facts about the Most Used and Abused Drugs from Alcohol to Ecstasy. (4th ed.). Cynthia Kuhn, Scott Swartzwelder, and Wilkie Wilson. Norton. 2014.

Drugs without the Hot Air: Minimising the Harms of Legal and Illegal Drugs. David Nutt. UIT Cambridge. 2012.

From Chocolate to Morphine: Everything You Need to Know about Mind-Altering Drugs. Andrew Weil and Winifred Rosen. Houghton Mifflin. 2004.

Illegal Drugs: A Complete Guide to Their History, Chemistry, Use, and Abuse. Paul Gahlinger. Sagebrush. 2001.

Julien's Primer of Drug Action: A Comprehensive Guide to the Actions, Uses, and Side Effects of Psychoactive Drugs (13th ed.). Claire Advokat, Joseph Comaty, Robert Julien. Worth. 2014.

Licit and Illicit Drugs: The Consumers Union Report on Narcotics, Stimulants, Depressants, Inhalants, Hallucinogens, and Marijuana—Including Caffeine, Nicotine, and Alcohol. Edward M. Brecher. Consumer Reports. 1973.

Out of It: A Cultural History of Intoxication. Stuart Walton. Three Rivers Press. 2002.

Street Drugs: A Drug Identification Guide, 2017. Publishers Group West. *www.streetdrugs.org.*

Uppers, Downers, All Arounders: Physical and Mental Effects of Psychoactive Drugs (8th ed.). Darryl Inaba and William Cohen. CNS Publications. 2014.

Websites

Drug Policy Alliance Drug Facts, *www.drugpolicy.org/drug-facts*

Drugs.com, *www.drugs.com* (for legal and illegal drugs)

Drugs Forum, *www.drugs-forum.com*

EROWID, *www.erowid.org*

Harm Reduction Coalition, *www.harmreduction.org*

Multidisciplinary Association for Psychedelic Studies, *www.maps.org*

National Organization for the Reform of Marijuana Laws, *www.norml.org*

Tweaker.org, *www.tweaker.org*

Substance Use, Substance Misuse, and Treatment: Theories, Research, and Critiques

Addiction: A Disorder of Choice. Gene M. Heyman. Harvard University Press. 2009.

"Addiction and Choice: Theory and New Data." Gene M. Heyman. *Frontiers in Psychiatry, 4,* 31. 2013.

"Adverse Childhood Experiences and the Association with Ever Using Alcohol and Initiating Alcohol Use During Adolescence." S. R. Dube et al. *Journal of Adolescent Health, 38*(4) 444.e1–444.e10. 2006.

Alcoholics Anonymous: Cult or Cure? Charles Bufe. See Sharp Press. 1991.

The Biology of Desire: Why Addiction Is Not a Disease. Marc Lewis. PublicAffairs. 2015.

"The Codependency Movement: Issues of Context and Differentiation." Judith R. Gordon and Kimberly Barrett. In John S. Baer, G. Alan Marlatt, and Robert J. McMahon, Eds. *Addictive Behaviors Across the Life Span: Prevention, Treatment, and Policy Issues.* SAGE. 1993.

Coming to Harm Reduction Kicking and Screaming: Looking for Harm Reduction in a 12-Step World. Dee-Dee Stout. AuthorHouse. 2009.

"Contemporary Psychoanalytic Theories of Substance Abuse: A Disorder in Search of a Paradigm." Jon Morgenstern and Jeremy Leeds. *Psychotherapy, 30,* 194–206. 1993.

Creating the Capacity for Attachment: Treating Addictions and the Alienated Self. Karen Walant. Jason Aronson. 1995.

The Disease Concept of Alcoholism. E. Morton Jellinek. Hillhouse Press. 1960.

Drugs, Behavior, and Modern Society (8th ed.). Charles Levinthal. Pearson. 2013.

Drug, Set, and Setting: The Basis for Controlled Intoxicant Use. Norman E. Zinberg. Yale University Press. 1984.

"Drug Use as a Protective System." L. Wurmser. In *Theories on Drug Abuse: Selected Contemporary Perspectives* (NIDA Monograph 30). Washington, DC: U.S. Department of Health and Human Services. 1980.

Harm Reduction Journal. www.harmreductionjournal.biomedcentral.com.

Harm Reduction: Pragmatic Strategies for Managing High-Risk Behaviors. G. Alan Marlatt, Mary E. Larimer, and Katie Witkiewitz, Eds. New York: Guilford Press. 1998.

Harm Reduction: Pragmatic Strategies for Managing High-Risk Behaviors (2nd ed.). G. Alan Marlatt, Mary E. Larimer, and Katie Witkiewitz, Eds. New York: Guilford Press. 2012.

Harm Reduction Psychotherapy: A New Treatment for Drug and Alcohol Problems. Andrew Tatarsky. Jason Aronson. 2002.

Heavy Drinking: The Myth of Alcoholism as a Disease. Herbert Fingarette. University of California Press. 1988.

High Price: A Neuroscientist's Journey of Self-Discovery That Challenges Everything You Know about Drugs and Society. Carl Hart. HarperCollins. 2013.

Hooked: Five Addicts Challenge Our Misguided Drug Rehab System. Lonny Shavelson. New Press. 2001.

"If at First You Don't Succeed: False Hopes of Self-Change." Janet Polivy and C. Peter Herman. *American Psychologist, 57*(9), 677–689. 2002.

I'm Dysfunctional, You're Dysfunctional: The Recovery Movement and Other Self-Help Fashions. Wendy Kaminer. Addison-Wesley. 1992.

Inside Rehab: The Surprising Truth about Addiction Treatment—And How to Get the Help That Works. Anne Fletcher. Viking. 2013

In the Realm of Hungry Ghosts: Close Encounters with Addiction. Gabor Mate. North Atlantic Books. 2010.

"The Likely Cause of Addiction Has Been Discovered, and It Is Not What You Think." Johann Hari. *Huffington Post,* January 20, 2015. *www.huffingtonpost.com/johann-hari/the-real-cause-of-addicti_b_6506936.html.*

Mindfulness-Based Relapse Prevention for Addictive Behaviors: A Clinician's Guide. Sarah Bowen, Neha Chawla, and G. Alan Marlatt. Guilford Press. 2011.

"Natural Recovery from Heroin Addiction: A Review of the Incidence Literature." Dan Waldorf and Patrick Biernacki. *Journal of Drug Issues,* 1979. *http://druglibrary.eu/library/articles/narehead.htm.*

Practicing Harm Reduction Psychotherapy: An Alternative Approach to Addictions (2nd ed.). Patt Denning and Jeannie Little. Guilford Press. 2012.

"Quitting Drugs: Quantitative and Qualitative Features." Gene M. Heyman. *Annual Review of Clinical Psychology, 9,* 29–59. 2013.

Relapse Prevention: Maintenance Strategies in the Treatment of Addictive Behaviors (2nd ed.). G. Alan Marlatt and Dennis M. Donovan, Eds. Guilford Press. 2005.

Rethinking Substance Abuse: What the Science Shows, and What We Should Do about It. William R. Miller and Kathleen M. Carroll, Eds. Guilford Press. 2006.

Seeking Safety: A Treatment Manual for PTSD and Substance Abuse. Lisa M. Najavits. Guilford Press. 2002.

"The Self-Medication Hypotheses of Addictive Disorders: Focus on Heroin and Cocaine Dependence." E. Khantzian. *American Journal of Psychiatry, 142,* 1259–1264. 1985.

The Sober Truth: Debunking the Bad Science behind 12-Step Programs and the Rehab Industry. Lance Dodes and Zachary Dodes. Beacon Press. 2014.

The Truth about Addiction and Recovery. Stanton Peele. Simon & Schuster. 1992. Up-to-date information at *www.peele.net.*

Unbroken Brain: A Revolutionary New Way of Understanding Addiction. Maia Szalavitz. St. Martin's Press. 2016.

Large-Scale Surveys of Drug Use Trends

Behavioral Health Trends in the United States: Results from the 2014 National Survey on Drug Use and Health (HHS Publication No. SMA 15-4927). Center for Behavioral Health Statistics and Quality. (2015). *www.samhsa.gov/data.*

Introduction to the National Epidemiological Survey of Alcohol and Related Conditions. Bridget F. Grant and Deborah A. Dawson. National Institute on Alcohol Abuse and Alcoholism. 2001/2002. *http://pubs.niaaa.nih.gov/publications/arh29-2/74-78.htm.*

Results from the 2013 National Survey on Drug Use and Health: Summary of National Findings (HHS Publication No. 14-4863). Substance Abuse and Mental Health Services Administration. 2014.

Related Theory and Research (Attachment, Trauma, Neurobiology, and Self-Determination)

Affect Regulation and the Origin of Self: The Neurobiology of Emotional Development. Allan N. Schore. Taylor & Francis. 1995.

The Body Keeps the Score: Brain, Mind, and Body in the Healing of Trauma. Bessel Van der Kolk. Penguin Books. 2014.

Brainwashed: The Seductive Appeal of Mindless Neuroscience. Sally Satel and Scot Lilienfeld. Basic Books. 2013.

Healing Trauma: Attachment, Mind, Body, and Brain. Marion F. Solomon and Daniel J. Siegel, Eds. Norton. 2003.

Motivational Interviewing: Helping People Change (3rd ed.). William R. Miller and Stephen Rollnick. Guilford Press. 2012.

Pocket Guide to Interpersonal Neurobiology: An Integrative Handbook of the Mind. Daniel Siegel. Norton. 2014.

A Secure Base: Parent–Child Attachment and Healthy Human Attachment. John Bowlby. Basic Books. 1988.

"Self-Determination Theory and the Facilitation of Intrinsic Motivation, Social Development, and Well-Being." R. Ryan and E. Deci. *American Psychologist, 55,* 68–78. 2000.

"Self-Determination Theory Applied to Health Contexts: A Meta-Analysis." J. Y. Y. Ng et al. *Perspectives on Psychological Science, 74*(4), 324–340. 2012.

Trauma and Recovery: The Aftermath of Violence, from Domestic Abuse to Political Terror. Judith Herman. Basic Books. 1997.

Drug Policy

Organizations

Break the Chains: Communities of Color and the War on Drugs

Canadian Harm Reduction Network, *www.canadianharmreduction.com*

Drug Policy Alliance, *www.drugpolicy.org*

Drug Reform Coordination Network, *www.stopthedrugwar.org*

Harm Reduction Australia, *www.harmreductionaustralia.org.au*

Harm Reduction Coalition, *www.harmreduction.org*

Harm Reduction International, *www.hri.global*

Law Enforcement Action Partnership (international organization), *www.leap.cc*

Midwest Harm Reduction Institute, *www.heartlandalliance.org/mhri*

Moms United to End the War on Drugs, *www.momsunited.net*

Open Society Foundations, *www.opensocietyfoundations.org*

The Sentencing Project, *www.sentencingproject.org*

Stop the Drug War, *www.stopthedrugwar.org*

Students for Sensible Drug Policy, *www.ssdp.org*

Drug Users' Unions

There are many around the world. For a listing, go to the International Network of People who Use Drugs: *www.inpud.net*

These are the largest in North America:

San Francisco Drug Users Union, *www.sfdrugusersunion.com*

Vancouver Area Network of Drug Users, *www.vandu.org*

VOCAL New York, *www.vocal-ny.org*

Books, Articles, and Reports

The American Disease: Origins of Narcotic Control. David Musto. Oxford University Press. 1987.

Caught in the Net: The Impact of Drug Policies on Women and Families. ACLU, Break the Chains, and the Brennan Center for Justice. *www.aclu.org.*

Chasing the Scream: The First and Last Days of the War on Drugs. Johann Hari. Bloomsbury. 2015.

Drug Crazy: How We Got into This Mess and How We Can Get Out. Mike Gray. Random House. 1998.

"Ethics and Drug Policy." Alex Wodak. *Psychiatry, 6*(2), 59–62. 2007.

The Globalization of Addiction: A Study in Poverty of the Spirit. Bruce K. Alexander. Oxford University Press. 2008.

"Harm Reduction Decade." Harm Reduction International. 2016. *www.hri.global/ harm-reduction-decade.*

"The Irrationality of Alcoholics Anonymous." Gabrielle Glaser. *The Atlantic,* April 2015. *www.theatlantic.com/magazine/archive/2015/04/the-irrationality-of-alcoholics-anonymous/386255.*

Last Call: The Rise and Fall of Prohibition. Daniel Okrent. Scribner. 2010.

Making Sense of Student Drug Testing: Why Educators are Saying No (2nd ed.) The ACLU and the Drug Policy Alliance (no date). *www.drugpolicy.org/docUploads/ drug_testing_booklet.pdf.*

The Narcotic Farm: The Rise and Fall of America's First Prison for Drug Addicts. Nancy D. Campbell, J. P. Olsen, and Luke Walden. Abrams. 2008.

The New Jim Crow: Mass Incarceration in the Age of Colorblindness. Michelle Alexander. New Press. 2012.

Nothing about Us Without Us—Greater, Meaningful Involvement of People Who Use Illegal Drugs: A Public Health, Ethical, and Human Rights Imperative. Open Society Institute with the Canadian HIV/AIDS Legal Network and International HIV/AIDS Alliance. 2008.

Films

The House I Live In. Eugene Jarecki. 2012.

For Families and Friends

Beyond Addiction: How Science and Kindness Help People Change. Jeffrey Foote, Carrie Wilkens, and Nicole Kosanke with Stephanie Higgs. Scribner. 2014.

Help at Any Cost: How the Troubled-Teen Industry Cons Parents and Hurts Kids. Maia Szalavitz. Riverhead Books. 2006.

Not My Family, Never My Child: What to Do If Someone You Love Is a Drug User. Tony Trimingham. Allen & Unwin. 2009. (Also the Stepping Stone workbook for families by Tony Trimingham.)

Safety First: A Reality-Based Approach to Teens and Drugs. Marsha Rosenbaum. PDFs available online in several languages. *www.drugpolicy.org/resource/safety-first-reality-based-approach-teens-and-drugs.*

Index

About the Authors

Patt Denning, PhD, is Director of Clinical Services and Training at the Center for Harm Reduction Therapy (CHRT) in San Francisco, which she founded with Jeannie Little in 2000. Widely recognized as an expert on drug treatment as well as treatment of other emotional and psychological issues, Dr. Denning is one of the principal developers of harm reduction psychotherapy.

Jeannie Little, LCSW, is Executive Director of CHRT. A certified group psychotherapist, Ms. Little was the first to implement harm reduction therapy in a group setting and has since adapted harm reduction therapy for widely diverse communities.

Together, Dr. Denning and Ms. Little are coauthors of a related book for mental health professionals, *Practicing Harm Reduction Psychotherapy, Second Edition.*